Web Health Information
Resource Guide

Web Health Information Resource Guide

For Consumers, Healthcare Providers, Patients and Physicians

Eugene A. DeFelice, M.D.

Authors Choice Press
San Jose New York Lincoln Shanghai

Web Health Information Resource Guide
For Consumers, Healthcare Providers, Patients and Physicians

Authors Choice Press
an imprint of iUniverse.com, Inc.

For information address:
iUniverse.com, Inc.
5220 S 16th, Ste. 200
Lincoln, NE 68512
www.iuniverse.com

ISBN: 0-595-19678-0

Printed in the United States of America

Dedication

This book is dedicated to my brother, Ben DeFelice, a literary agent, world traveler, raconteur extraordinaire, and friend and helping hand to many, who is now fortunate to be enjoying retirement with a number of his many friends. He enlisted in the Maritime Service in World War II, answering the call of duty early in the hostilities. Ben repeatedly volunteered for, and engaged in, a number of dangerous missions for his country and the benefit and good of others without regard for his own life and safety, and is regarded by all who know him as a "true patriot and man of all seasons". As one who has done so much for so many, as well as his Country, his life example has inspired me to write this book in the hope that it also, will touch the lives of many others and help them to enjoy a more productive, healthier, happier and longer life

Contents

Dedication v

Preface ix

Acknowledgements xiii

Chapter I Health Overview 1

    Your Health/Your Responsibility: Healthy People 2010 ....*1*

    Leading Causes of Death in the United States *3*

    Abortions *4*

    Alcohol, Drug Abuse and Health *5*

    Tobacco and Health *6*

    Physical Activity and Health and Obesity *7*

    Nutrition and Health and Obesity *9*

    Medical and Surgical Errors and Health *11*

    Influenza and Pneumonia *13*

    Accidents *13*

    Mental Health, Disability, and Suicide *13*

    Reduction in Leading Causes of Death *14*

    Healthy Life Style *14*

    Table III-Principles Which Contribute to a Healthy Life Style *14*

Chapter II World Wide Web and Internet 17

    World Wide Web *17*

    Internet *17*

    Browsers *18*

    Search Engine, Directory, Index, and WebCrawler *18*

    URL, Scheme, Domain Name and Zone *18*

    MeSH Term *20*

Chapter III Web Health Information Search Tools 22

    Introduction *22*

    Search Engines, Directories, Indexes, Meta Search Engines: Similarities and Differences *23*

Search Engines *24*

Directories *24*

Indexes *24*

Hybrids *25*

Meta Search Engines *25*

Overview *26*

Recommended Search Engines (University of California at Berkley) *27*

Recommended Subject Directories (University of California at Berkley) ..*28*

Recommended Meta Search Engines (University of California at Berkeley) 28

Recommended Search Tools (National Network of Libraries of Medicine) 29

Recommended Search Tools (Search Engine Databases and Newswires) *29*

Selected Popular Major Search Engines Directories and Indexes *30*

Selected US Government Search Tools *34*

Medical Colleges, Universities and Hospital Medical Centers *35*

Chapter IV Author's List of Selected Useful Search Tools and Web Sites *36*

Chapter V Health Categories, Diseases, Resources, and Web Sites ..114

Chapter VI Health Resources and Web Sites 243

Chapter VII Search the Internet/Web for Health Information 267

About the Author 271

Preface

Vast numbers of people in the Western World, particularly the United States, tend to

> Squander health in search of wealth,
> They work, and toil and save
> Then squander wealth in search of health
> But find an early grave.
>
> Anonymous

The majority of people tend to pay little or no attention to a healthy lifestyle or their health and wellness. They tend to "live their lives backwards" so to speak, per the example above, and thus suffer the consequences.

Most of us need to change our lifestyle for the better, become knowledgeable and do what is best for our health and wellness. The Internet and Web provides easily accessible information and ways to accomplish these goals and objectives. The name of the game is "you bet your life" and the Internet and Web may help you to improve your health and wellness, prolong your life span and perhaps even to save your life. So become involved and knowledgeable about your health and wellness, and healthcare and profit accordingly.

It is now widely recognized that-

> Healthcare is not what it used to be
> Healthcare is not even what it ought to be
> Health information on the Web seems destined to be
> Health information available for all as it should be
>
> Eugene A. De Felice, M.D.

This book provides the means at your fingertips, to quickly and easily search the Internet and Web and obtain the best, current health information that you can use to transform your life. With such information, you can take charge, control, and responsibility for your health, wellness and healthcare and make informed decisions with your physician or healthcare providers for your betterment. Should you not be satisfied with your healthcare provider, treatment or facility, you can use Web health information to intelligently voice your concern and opinion, and obtain better healthcare elsewhere if need be. In this way you may not only help to improve your own health and healthcare but also play an important role in transforming the healthcare system for the better for all concerned.

Your health and wellness and healthcare depends largely on the:

- Place where you live;
- Healthcare facility in which you are treated;
- Training, experience, knowledge and proficiency of your physician or healthcare provider;
- Degree to which you become well enough informed to take charge, control, and responsibility for your health, wellness and healthcare and make informed decisions; and
- Healthcare plan under which you receive treatment.

The healthcare information you receive, diagnosis made and treatment given for any disease or condition you may have, not only varies greatly among physicians in any given community, but also from facility to facility across the United States and throughout the Western World. Unfortunately, misuse, overuse, and under use of healthcare is much more common than one might presume. Many medical, surgical, psychological or psychiatric practices are not evidence based but rather dependent on unproven methods, fads, anecdotal information or even speculation, and not uncommonly used without the patient's knowledge or consent. Today, physicians may even find themselves "too busy" or "not knowledgeable enough" to fully explain treatment, options, and outcomes and obtain true informed consent from the patient. In this age of managed care and the "business" of medical care, HMOs and other practices not uncommonly tend to be more concerned with the "bottom line". As a result, the best treatment may not even be offered to the patient because of cost or other reasons. All of this is not in the best interests of the patient. Therefore, patients must take charge, control, and responsibility for their health, wellness and healthcare and change things for the better and to live a healthier, happier, longer and more enjoyable life.

This book is organized into 7 chapters. Chapter I provides a Health Overview on a number of relevant health topics. Chapter II briefly outlines essentials of the Web and the Internet. Chapter III discusses a variety of Web Health Search Tools. The Author's List of 70 key Selected Useful Search Tools and Web sites as well as an outline of health, wellness and healthcare information contained in each is reviewed in Chapter IV. An alphabetical list of over 100 key Health Categories with corresponding Diseases and Conditions, Health Information Resources, and Web sites for each is contained in Chapter V to help facilitate searching the Web for health information. Chapter VI provides an alphabetical list of over 300 Health and Wellness Resources and their corresponding Web sites reviewed for this book. Chapter VII (as well as Chapters III and VI) contains useful suggestions for optimizing searching the Web for health, wellness and healthcare information. The Table of Contents provides a more detailed outline of each chapter and subdivision.

Time Magazine June 4, 2001, vol. 157, no. 22, page 25 states that 100 million Americans consult the Internet/Web for health information and 70% say the information they find influences treatment decisions. This book is designed to greatly facilitate your obtaining and using such health, wellness and healthcare information.

Acknowledgements

Special appreciation is given to Ms. Maryanne Harvey, for her knowledge, competence, inspiration, dedication and care in helping to prepare and edit the manuscript for this book for publication. Without her friendship, encouragement and able assistance this book would not have been possible.

Chapter I

Health Overview

Your Health/Your Responsibility: Healthy People 2010

Government agencies are primarily responsible for the health of the general public, for people as a group. The US Government program "Healthy People 2010: Priority Areas of Healthcare Focus Areas" is outlined in Table I. Governmental actions in the priority focus areas are regarded as essential for improving the public health in general.

Table I-Healthy People 2010 Focus Areas

- Access to Quality Health Services
- Arthritis, Osteoporosis, and Chronic Back Conditions
- Cancer
- Chronic Kidney Disease
- Diabetes
- Disability and Secondary Conditions
- Educational and Community Based Programs
- Environmental Health
- Family Planning
- Food Safety

- Health Communication
- Heart Diseases and Stroke
- HIV
- Immunization and Infectious Disease
- Injury and Violence Prevention
- Maternal, Infant and Child Health
- Medical Product Safety
- Mental Health and Mental Disorders
- Nutrition and Overweight
- Occupational Safety and Health
- Oral Health
- Physical Activity and Fitness
- Public Health Infrastructure
- Respiratory Diseases
- Sexually Transmitted Diseases
- Substance Abuse
- Tobacco Use
- Vision and Hearing

"Healthy People 2010" is a national health promotion and disease prevention initiative that brings together national, state, and local government agencies, non-profit, voluntary and professional organizations, businesses, communities, and individuals to improve the health of all Americans, eliminate disparities in health, and extend and improve quality of life. The 1979 Surgeon General's Report, "Healthy People and Healthy People 2000: National Health Promotion and Disease Prevention Objectives", both established national health objectives and served as the basis for the development of state and community plans. The new "Healthy People 2010" goals and objectives were launched on January 25, 2000.

"Healthy People 2010" builds on initiatives pursued over the past two decades and will be monitored through 467 objectives in 28 focus areas (outlined in Table I) designed to reduce or eliminate illness, disability and premature death among individuals and communities. Others focus on broader issues, such as improving access to quality healthcare, strengthening public health services and improving availability and dissemination of health related information. Each objective has a target for specific improvement to be achieved by the year 2010. For this and further information on Healthy People 2000 and 2010 programs the reader is referred to:

http://www.health.gov/healthypeople

However, the aforementioned government programs will not directly improve your own personal health; they will do so only indirectly at best. You and your physician or healthcare provider are the ones primarily concerned with you as an individual. Both of you are responsible for your health, wellness and healthcare. Your physician or healthcare provider is in the best position to help you achieve or maintain your own personal good health and provide you with the best of healthcare should you become ill. However, in the final analysis, it should be recognized that your health, wellness and healthcare is largely up to you since you may control well over two thirds of the factors involved in your health status. So be governed accordingly and become responsible, informed and involved.

Leading Causes of Death in the United States

Table II provides estimated figures for the leading causes of death in the United States adapted from figures obtained from the Centers for Disease Control and Prevention (http://www.cdc.gov), the Agency for Healthcare Research and Quality (http://www.ahrq.gov), the National Institute on Alcohol Abuse and Alcoholism (http://www.niaaa.nih.gov), and the National Institute on Drug Abuse (http://www.nida.nih.gov) as well as the author's own estimates derived from a variety of sources.

Table II-Estimated Figures for Leading Causes of Death in the United States *

- Abortion — ~ 1,500,000
- Heart disease — ~750,000
- Cancer — ~500,000
- Obesity** — ~150,000
- Stroke — ~150,000
- Alcohol/Drug Abuse — ~130,000
- COPD*** — ~100,000
- Medical/surgical errors — ~95,000
- Accidents **** — ~90,000
- Pneumonia and influenza — ~85,000
- Diabetes — ~60,000
- Suicide — ~30,000
- Kidney disease — ~25,000
- Liver disease — ~25,000
- Fire arms and murder — ~15,000

*approximations only (to show orders of magnitude)
**author's estimate from a variety of sources (likely underestimated)
***chronic obstructive pulmonary disease
****auto ~40,000, other ~50,000

Abortions

Most abortions are elective and preventable via proper family planning, birth control measures, and adoption. Emotional and other mental disorders suffered by the mother who undergoes an abortion also are preventable. Thus, abortion remains as a key focus of attention in terms of reducing the death and disability rate in the United States.

Alcohol, Drug Abuse and Health

Ten percent of adults, including young adults, in the United States may be classified today as problem drinkers, alcohol abusers, or alcoholics who have experienced the negative consequences of alcohol use at some time in their life. The adverse public health consequences of drinking alcohol are numerous and include among other things:

- Abuse (family, others)
- Accidents (home, motor vehicle, work)
- Crime and incarceration
- Injuries, disability, impaired health
- Premature death
- Impaired mental and emotional health
- Violence and its consequences

An estimated one third to one half of all unintentionally or intentionally injured adult or young adult Americans involved in accidents, crimes, homicide, or suicide are reported to have been drinking alcohol. Problem drinking also causes extensive damage to health including such things as pancreatitis, nutritional deficiencies, malignancies, fetal alcohol syndrome, and cirrhosis (one of the leading causes of death among adults in the United States).

The National Institute on Drug Abuse (http://www.nida.nih.gov) along with the National Institute on Alcohol Abuse and Alcoholism (http://www.niaaa.nih.gov) published a report entitled "The Economic Costs of Alcohol and Drug Abuse in the United States 1992". In this report, it is estimated that in 1992, more than 132,000 persons died prematurely as a consequence of alcohol and drug problems. Of these, 107,400 were related to alcohol abuse and 25,500 to drug abuse. Many of the alcohol and drug related deaths occurred among persons between 20 and 40 years of age because the major causes of death, such as motor vehicle crashes, other causes of traumatic death and HIV infection, are concentrated among younger age cohorts. However, alcohol is also involved in numerous premature deaths among the older population because of long-term, excessive alcohol consumption. Also, it was estimated that in 1995, alcohol abuse cost $166.5 billion and drug abuse, $109.8 billion. These costs were attributed principally to premature deaths, impaired productivity, motor vehicle crashes, crime and other causes. Thus, minimizing alcohol intake and abstaining from illegal drugs are two key ways to promote a healthy life style and help reduce death and disability from these two sources.

Tobacco and Health

The National Center for Chronic Disease Prevention and Health Promotion (NCCDPHP) estimates that, in the United States, tobacco use results in:

- About 430,000 deaths attributable to cigarette smoking each year (smoking is reported to cause up to 90% of all lung cancer and cessation significantly reduces deaths from lung cancer).
- Direct medical costs associated with smoking of more then $50 billion or about 7% of the total cost of healthcare in the United States in 1997.
- Approximately one of every two lifelong smokers eventually dies of smoking related illness.
- An estimated 25 million persons alive today, including 5 million children younger than 18 years of age, will die prematurely of smoking attributable diseases
- About 10 million people in the United States have died of smoking attributable causes (including lung and other cancers, emphysema, other respiratory diseases and heart disease) since the first Surgeon • General Report on Smoking and Health in 1964

To further back up these statistics, the NCCDPHP site provides reports on:

- Chronic Disease and Their Risk Factors: the Nation's Leading Cause of Death
- Guidelines for School Health Programs to Prevent Tobacco Use and Addiction
- State and National Tobacco Control Highlights
- Targeting Tobacco Use: The Nation's Leading Cause of Death At-A-Glance
- CDC's Tips: Tobacco Information and Prevention Source

Further information on this subject is available from the National Center for Chronic Disease Prevention and Health promotion:

http://cdc.gov/nccdph/tobacco.htm

Stopping smoking is a "must" for good health and reducing unnecessary deaths and disability from tobacco related disease.

Physical Activity and Health and Obesity

According to the Centers for Disease Control and Prevention, millions of Americans suffer from illnesses that can be prevented through regular physical activity. CDC estimates that:

- 13.5 million people have coronary heart disease
- 1.5 million people suffer from a heart attack in a given year
- 8 million plus people have adult onset (non-insulin dependent) diabetes mellitus
- 95,000 people are newly diagnosed with colon cancer each year
- over 60 million people (a quarter of the population) are overweight

A recent report entitled "Physical Activity and Health: A Report of the Surgeon General" brings together for the first time what has been learned about physical activity and health from decades of research. Among its major findings are:

- People who are usually inactive can improve their health and reduce the risks of obesity and developing or dying from, heart disease, diabetes, high blood pressure and colon cancer by becoming even moderately active on a regular basis
- Physical activity need not be strenuous to achieve health benefits and still greater health benefits can be achieved by increasing the amount of physical activity
- Inactivity increases with age and is more common among women and those with lower income and less education
- Nearly half of young people aged 12-21 years are not vigorously active on a regular basis. More than 60% of adults do not achieve the recommended amount of regular physical activity. In fact, 25% of all adults are not active at all.

CDC points out that in older adults:

- Loss of strength and stamina attributed to aging is, in part, caused by reduced activity
- Inactivity increases with age. By age 75, about one in three men and one in two women engage in no physical activity.
- Among adults aged 65 and older, walking and gardening or yard work are, by far, the most popular physical activities
- Social support from family and friends has been consistently and positively related to regular physical activity

And physical activity is reported to benefit senior citizens as well in the following ways:

- Helps maintain the ability to live independently and reduces the risk of falling and fractures

- Reduces the risk of dying from coronary heart disease, high blood pressure, stroke, colon cancer, and diabetes
- Helps to reduce blood pressure in patients with hypertension promoting better control of blood pressure
- Helps people with chronic, disabling conditions improve their stamina and muscle strength
- Reduces symptoms of anxiety and depression and fosters improvement in mood and well-being
- Helps to maintain healthy bones, muscles, and joints, and prevent osteoporosis
- Helps to control joint swelling and pain associated with arthritis.

Further information on physical activity and health can be obtained via National Center for Chronic Disease Prevention and Health promotion web sites:

> http://www.cdc.gov/nccdphp/phyactive.htm
> http://www.cdc.gov/nccdphp/sgr/mm.htm

Nutrition and Health and Obesity

Obesity is now believed to be one of the leading causes of death in the United States and Western World. Obesity has now reached epidemic proportions in the United States and poor nutrition is rampant.

In a report on the "Impact of Nutrition on Health", the Centers for Disease Control and Prevention states that improving the American diet could extend productive life spans and reduce the occurrence of chronic disease, including cardiovascular disease, cancer and diabetes. It also concludes that:

- Poor diet and physical inactivity are associated with 300,000 unnecessary deaths each year, second only to tobacco use;

- Of all adult Americans, 52% are overweight or obese (i.e., have a body mass index of 25 or greater) and 21% are obese (i.e., have a body mass index of 30 or greater);
- Obesity contributes to a variety of diseases, including heart disease, diabetes, and cancer. In the United States alone, the economic cost of obesity approximates 100 billion (in 1995 dollars) annually; and
- One half of adult Americans have cholesterol levels above the desired 200 milligrams/dl.

The National Center for Chronic Disease Prevention and Health Promotion (http://www.cdc.gov/nccdphp/nutrisk.htm) provides further information on the impact of nutrition and obesity on health as well as reports on:

- Guidelines for School Health Programs to Promote Lifelong Healthy Eating
- CDC's Nutrition and Physical Activity Program

Risk factors such as obesity, sedentary, unhealthy life style, poor nutrition, high blood pressure and smoking may lead to heart attacks, vascular disease, diabetes, kidney disease and stroke increasing the death rate and disability from these disorders. Controlling and reducing such risk factors decreases corresponding death/disabilities rates. For example, it is estimated that over 50% of deaths from heart disease are preventable by controlling risk factors alone. Proper nutrition, diet and exercise and weight control also significantly reduce the death and disability rate and improves health and well being and needs to be a priority area of interest and action for all.

Medical and Surgical Errors and Health

Medical or surgical treatment not uncommonly is based on unreliable information and may be administered without the patient's knowledge or consent. Serious errors may occur as a result. Thus, the patient needs to become aware and informed about evidenced based options and outcomes. The Dartmouth Atlas of Health Care (http://www. dartmouthatlas.org) is a good place to start.

Medical and Surgical errors as a group are one of the leading causes of death and injury in the United States. The National Academy of Sciences Institute of Medicine (http://www.iom.edu) and Agency for Healthcare Research and Quality (http://www.ahrq.gov/qual/errors.htm) estimate that up to 100,000 people die each year in US hospitals as a result of medical and surgical errors. The true figure may be even higher in this writer's estimation, particularly if outpatient deaths are included. As one can see from Table II, "Estimated Figures for Leading Causes of Death in the United States", more people are reported to die from medical and surgical errors in hospitals or other healthcare facilities than from accidents, pneumonia and influenza, breast cancer, diabetes, suicide, kidney disease, or liver disease. Government agencies, health care providers, and others are working to improve the safety of the US healthcare system. As a patient, you also can do your part by becoming involved not only for your own sake but also for others by helping to improve the healthcare system.

Medical and surgical errors occur in all parts of the healthcare system: clinics, doctor's offices, hospitals, nursing homes, outpatient surgery or emergency centers, pharmacies, and even in patient's homes. And errors may involve doctor's or nurse's reports, equipment, diagnosis, lab studies or reports, surgery or treatment. Thus, as a patient and consumer, you must be informed and vigilant at all times and in all places in order to help reduce such errors.

The complexity of the healthcare system itself fosters many problems which can result in errors. At times, the "left hand dyskinesia syndrome" prevails: in other words, the left hand does not know what the right is doing, communication is poor, and not uncommonly medical and surgical care is not well coordinated, resulting in suboptimal care and worse. Today's busy physicians and healthcare providers not uncommonly fail to find the time to help patients become knowledgeable and make informed decisions. And poorly informed and involved patients are less likely to understand, accept, or follow their physician's advice and treatment. As such, patients are less likely to do what is necessary to help make any given treatment successful.

Thus, the single most important way you can help to insure that you receive the best and most appropriate medical and surgical care and prevent errors is to become an active, involved and informed member of your health care team. While you can do this in a variety of ways, especially through your physician or health care provider, the Internet and Web also provides one of the better ways to accomplish this goal. For 20 tips on how to help prevent medical and surgical errors by becoming an active, informed member of your healthcare team, consult the Agency for Healthcare Research and Quality:

http://www.ahrq.gov/consumer/20tips.htm.

You can obtain additional information on each of these 20 tip areas by searching the Web.

For further information on the impact of medical errors, consult: http://ww.iom.edu and type in "To Err is Human: Building a Safer Health System" under Search. Go to item 2 of 51 and click on Executive Summary, pp 1-16 for details. Go to: http://www.americanshealth.org and click on report entitled "Reducing Medical Errors and Improving Patient Safety, Released Feb. 22, 2000."

Influenza and Pneumonia

The majority of cases of influenza are preventable via a healthy life style and proper nutrition, immunization and hygiene. See various Web resources for vaccines and immunization schedules and ways to prevent death and disability from influenza and pneumonia.

Accidents

Buckle up your seat belt, avoid driving when tired or sleepy, drive carefully and defensively, and safely, and take the necessary measures to avoid accidents at work, home, or play. Avoid illegal drugs and limit the use of alcohol. In these ways, death and disability from accidents also can be reduced dramatically.

Mental Health, Disability, and Suicide

Anxiety and depression are common emotional problems of every day living and may become overwhelming. Both mental and physical well being may be affected. Prolonged anxiety and depression can ruin good health and precipitate disability, physical and/or mental disease. Live a healthy life style, reduce stress, enjoy the spiritual aspects of life, and meditate. These are ways to reduce anxiety, and depression and mental and emotional problems of everyday living. If you feel anxiety or depression may be a problem, consult the Web for information and help, and discuss the matter with your physician or healthcare provider, particularly if suicide is being considered.

Reduction in Leading Causes of Death

Abortion is a largely preventable leading cause of death. By becoming physically active and fit, improving your nutrition, reducing and abstaining from alcohol intake, avoiding illegal drugs, and tobacco and adopting a healthy life style will go a long way towards significantly reducing death and disability from leading causes of premature death discussed previously.

Healthy Life Style

In the final analysis, the best prescription for good health is to use your own good common sense, "listen" to your body and mind, and take charge, control, and responsibility for your health, wellness and healthcare and adopt a healthy life style. Among the principles which contribute to a healthy life style are practices such as those summarized in Table III.

Table III-Principles Which Contribute to a Healthy Life Style

- Alcohol use: sparingly or not at all
- Be a friend to many and have many friends
- Believe and have confidence in yourself
- Choose a physician and health care facility prudently
- Communicate effectively with family, friends, colleagues, and your physician or healthcare provider
- Comprehensive annual check-up
- Develop and maintain a rich and full spiritual life
- Discover your potential in life
- Do good
- Do no intentional harm to yourself or any thing
- Do not procrastinate: learn how to make decisions

- Drugs: abstain from illegal drugs and use prescription drugs only as recommended
- Eat in healthy and nutritionally sound ways
- Exercise and become physically fit
- Follow safety rules and avoid injuries
- Follow your bliss
- Have a laudable purpose in life
- Maintain good family relationships
- Make the world a better place
- Moderation in living, working and playing and avoid excesses
- Oral hygiene regularly
- Practice regularly and faithfully
    - Compassion
    - Forgiveness
    - Goodness
    - Joy
    - Justice
    - Love
    - Mercy
    - Patience
    - Peace
    - Self-control
    - Understanding
- Regular and restful sleep
- Relaxation and stress reduction daily
- Rest regularly
- Safe sexual practices
- Set and accomplish goals
- Strive for emotional well being and control
- Take charge, control, and responsibility for your health and life
- Tobacco use: not at all
- Weight control: attain and maintain ideal weight

The Web provides a great deal of information on how to achieve a healthy life style along the lines suggested on Table III. Search for further information on "healthy life style", and "take charge of your health", "take control of your health", and "take responsibility for your health", via the following web sites:

- American Academy of Family Physicians   http: //www.aafp.org
- American Medical Association   http: //www.ama-assn.org
- Healthfinder.gov   http://www.healthfinder.gov
- Yahoo.com   http://www.yahoo.com/health

Chapter II

World Wide Web and Internet

World Wide Web

The World Wide Web (www) is reported to have been invented by Tom Berners-Lee at the European Particle Physics Lab in Geneva, Switzerland in 1989. Berners-Lee has served as a Director of the World Wide Web Consortium (W3). He also is regarded as the inventor of HTTP (Hypertext Transport Protocol), the computer language in which pages on the Web are written.

Internet

The Internet is all the computers that are connected together into a global network so that they may communicate with each other. The Internet and the Web are not the same thing. The Internet started out in 1969 as a network of networks of computers. On the other hand, the Web commenced in 1989 as a system of interconnected information on computers in the form of Web pages that you access via the Internet.

Browsers

Browsers are software programs that let your computer show you pages of information on the Web. Netscape Navigator, Microsoft Internet Explorer, and AOL Browser are three of the most commonly used browsers.

Search Engine, Directory, Index, and WebCrawler

A Search Engine, Directory, Index, or Web Crawler, are different kinds of search tools that enable you to find pages of information on the Web regarding specific healthcare topics of interest to you.

URL, Scheme, Domain Name and Zone

URL (Uniform Resource Locator), the address code used to identify Web pages and most of the other information on the Web. URLs are standardized ways of naming resources and their Web addresses used for linking pages on the Web. A typical URL, for example, is the one for the Librarians' Index to the Internet which is written as:

http://www.lii.org

The first letters before the colon is called the "scheme" which describes the way a browser can get to the resource information. Although some ten "schemes" have been defined, the most common one in use is "http" which stands for hypertext language. Following http:// is www which stands for World Wide Web and then the "Domain Name" (host computer), namely lii, or Librarians' index to the Internet on which the information resides.

In searching the Web it is not always necessary to use the designations http:// www. Just the domain name and what comes after the dot (i.e., org) usually suffices.

Domain names in the United States usually end with three letters which are called the "zone" and provide a clue as to what kind of address it may be. Commercial organizations end with .com, educational with .edu, networking organizations with .net, US Government with a .gov and organizations that don't fall into any of those categories with an .org. Outside the United States, domain names usually end with a country code such as .ca for Canada, .ch for Switzerland, .it for Italy, .se for Sweden or .uk for United Kingdom.

Table IV summarizes the zone designations for Web sites used in this book.

Table IV-Selected domain Site Designations/Significance

Designation	Significance
.ca	Canada
.ch	Switzerland
.co.uk United Kingdom.	Use of .co implies site is commercial or miscellaneous
.com	mostly commercial
.edu	educational, mostly colleges and universities in North America
.gov	US Government
.it	Italy
.net	originally for networks but now also available for companies and individuals
.org	organization or association originally but now also available to companies and individuals
.se	Sweden

Generally speaking, health, wellness and healthcare information is considered to be more reliable on a .gov or .edu Web site compared with .org or .com sites. However, it should be remembered that this depends a great deal on the posting standards of the particular agency, institution, organization or commercial site involved. A number of .org, .com or country sites also provide high quality informational content, i.e., http://www.mic.ki.se (Karolinska Institutet of Sweden); hon.ch (Health on the Net Foundation of Switzerland); http: //www.irfmn.mnegri.it (Instituto Mario Negri of Italy), and http://www.herts.ac.uk (University of Hertsfordshire, United Kingdom). Keeping these basics in mind will help you in selecting appropriate search tools and Web sites and sifting through search results when credibility in health and wellness matters.

MeSH Term

MeSH (medical search term) is a vocabulary of medical and scientific terms assigned to documents in PubMed, Health on the Net, Karolinska Institute, or other search tools by a team of experts. These terms can be used in many cases to search more efficiently than simple text words.

MeSH terms may be assigned to the entire article with some being designated the major topic. Some MeSh terms may have subheadings and others even additional subheadings. In the search, MeSH terms are exploded which means that a search using a MeSH term finds not only documents indexed under the term, but also all documents indexed with more specific terms that are included in the meaning of the MeSH term used. Such an explosion is accomplished by use of a MeSH tree arrangement. For more information on MeSH terms definitions, go to: PubMed (National Library of Medicine):

http://www.ncbi.nlm.nih.gov/PubMed/meshbrowserhelp.html

For further basic information on learning the Internet and Web, the anatomy of a URL, domain names, Web pages, Web sites and Web browsers, the reader is referred to Learn the Net:

http://www.learnthenet.com

Chapter III

Web Health Information Search Tools

Introduction

Not all health, wellness, and healthcare information on the Web can be considered to be useful or reliable. Neither can the search tools and resources used to search the Web. Selectivity and due diligence on the part of the reader are a "must".

Health, wellness and healthcare information varies widely in scope, depth, usefulness, and reliability depending on the search tool(s) and Web site(s) or resource(s) used to obtain it. Therefore, it is important to use reliable guidelines when choosing these Web resources. Also, your search can be greatly improved by spending time learning the nuances of several search tools in order to choose the best ones for you and your purposes. Search engines do key word and topic searches against a database but various factors influence results such as size of database, frequency of update, search capability and design and speed. All these factors may lead to greatly different results.

Useful guidelines for evaluating Web sites and search tools can be obtained from certain Web sources, namely:

- American Medical Association: http://www.ama-assn.org/about-guidelines.htm
- Healthfinder: http://www.healthfinder.gov
- Health on the Net: http://www.hon.ch

The guidelines and criteria used by each of these organizations, as well as others, varies. Nevertheless, by using these resources and guidelines suggested above, or others, you should be better able to evaluate useful Web sites and search tools.

The Web is currently estimated at well over 1.5 billion pages and growing rapidly and is not indexed by any standard vocabulary as one finds in libraries. Therefore, when you search the Web, you are not searching it directly as this is not feasible at this time. The Web is the totality of the many millions upon millions of Web pages which reside on computers (called servers) worldwide and your computer cannot locate or search them directly. All you can do through your computer is to go to one of a number of intermediate databases which contain selected and organized Web pages and databases. Thus, you merely search the "intermediate search tools" and they provide you with links to other Web pages needed for your search. You can then click on these links and retrieve documents, etc. from individual servers (computers) around the world for the information you desire.

Search Engines, Directories, Indexes, Meta Search Engines: Similarities and Differences

There are a number of similarities and differences in search tools. Some of these similarities and differences are as follows.

Search Engines

Search Engines allow you to search the Web using key words to find relevant health, wellness and healthcare information on the Internet electronically and mechanically using "robots" and "spiders" and not people. They create databases of Web documents. These databases are created by programs called "spiders", "worms" or "bots". These programs roam the Web jumping from one URL to another indexing the Web page and adding it to the database in a mechanical fashion based on a specific pre-arranged formula and without any human intervention. Each search engine has its own formula for indexing pages, some index the whole site while others only the main page. The amount and kind of information you retrieve varies significantly from one search engine to another and results may represent the excellent, the good, the fair and the bad. Thus you must carefully evaluate all information you find before you believe or use it.

Directories

Directories are completely different from Search Engines. They use human indexing with people (not mechanical spiders and robots) reviewing and indexing links. People involved follow strict guidelines before adding information to their index. Thus, the human expert compiled indexed directory of health information generally can be considered to be more reliable and to the point, bearing in mind that some "experts" may be better than others in doing their job.

Indexes

An index, on the other hand, simply collects all items of information from the Web related to your search, extracts key words, and makes a large list. You then search the index list by specifying some words that seem likely to narrow the search, and the search tool you are using finds all the entries which contain that word(s). Because indexes are created largely or completely automatically, they are not selective and usually contain many more entries of information than you want. In contrast, once you find a category of information in a directory, all the items of information contained therein are likely to be related to what you want.

Hybrids

Hybrid commercial search engines combine a directory and a search engine and even indexes, and represent the new generation in use today. Yahoo, for example, is a directory which employs Google (a search engine) for its results. And Google uses Open Directory to supplement its own search engine.

Some overlap exists between indexes and directories as well. Yahoo lets you search by key word, and many of the indexes divide their entries into general categories that let you limit your search.

Meta Search Engines

These search tools use metasearch sites or metacrawlers that send out searches to several other different search engines and their databases of web pages. Meta search engines do not own their own databases of web pages and they spend only a short time searching other's databases. As a result, they often retrieve only around 10% of the information in any of the databases queried. This tends to make meta search engine searches more "quick and dirty" and not necessarily thorough and more useful. Thus, meta search engines should be used cautiously in interpreting results obtained.

Overview

More detailed information on the pros and cons and merits of these different types of search tools may be obtained from the following Web references:

- Search Engines: http://www.searchengines.com/search_engines.101.html
- Recommended Search Engines (University of California at Berkely): http://www.lib.berkley.edu/TeachingLib/Guides/Internet/Search_Engines.html
- Recommended Subject Directories (University of California at Berkely): http://www.lib.berkley.edu/TeachingLib/Guides/Internet/MetaSearch.html
- Recommended Meta Search Engines (University of California at Berkely): http://www.lib.berkley.edu/TeachingLib/Guides/Internet/SubjDirectories.html
- Recommended Search Tools (University of California at Berkley): http://www.lib.berkley.edu/TeachingLib/Guides/Internet/ToolsTables.html

Chapters III and IV of this book provide a description of the health information contained in each of the selected search tools considered by the author and others to be among the more useful for obtaining health-care information from the Web and thus are highlighted in this book.

Recommended Search Engines (University of California at Berkley)

The University of California at Berkley recommends 5 commercial Search Engines which they believe to be particularly useful. They are listed in Table V below and are included in the Author's List of Selected Useful Search Tools and Web Sites reviewed in Chapter IV of this book.

Table V Recommended Search Engines (University of California at Berkley)

- Alta Vista: Health Web Directory   dr.altavista.com/top/health
- Fast Search   fastsearch.com
  alltheweb.com
- Google Web Directory: Health   directory.google.com/top/health
- Infoseek Health and Wellness   infoseek.go.com/center/health
- Northern Light Search   northernlight.com

The http://www. prefix which normally appears before each of the domain names above has been omitted for brevity and clarity from this table. Use of http://www is not necessary to be employed in going to any one of the above Web sites. Only the domain name and zone need be used. This rule also pertains to the other tables which follows.

For the pros and cons and further information on these commercial Search Engines consult:

http://www.lib.berkley.edu/TeachingLib/Guides/Internet/Search_Engines.html

Recommended Subject Directories (University of California at Berkley)

Three commercial Subject Directories, covered in this book, are recommended as particularly useful by the University of California at Berkley are listed in Table VI.

Table VI Recommended Subject Directories (University of California at Berkley)

- About.com   about.com
- Librarian's Index   lii.org
- Yahoo   yahoo.com

For pros and cons and further information on these Subject Directories and others consult information provided in this book on each and:

http://www.lib.berkley.edu/TeachingLib/Guides/Internet/SubjDirectories.html

Recommended Meta Search Engines (University of California at Berkeley)

MetaCrawler is an example of a commercial MetaSearch Engine recommended by the University of California at Berkley Teaching Library. It is considered to be one of the best available. For further information on MetaCrawler and other Meta Search Engines consult:

http://www.lib.berkley.edu/TeachingLib/Guides/Internet/MetaSearch.html

The University of California at Berkley site recommends that since search engines and subject directories cited are "hand-selected", you should consult more than one for desired information on any given healthcare topic of interest.

Recommended Search Tools (National Network of Libraries of Medicine)

Six key search tools are recommended as useful for consumer health information by the national Network of libraries of medicine. For further information on these, consult:

http://www.nnlm.nlm.nih.gov/psr

A further description of these six key search tools can be found in Chapter III under National network of Libraries of Medicine.

Recommended Search Tools (Search Engine Databases and Newswires)

Features a collection of proprietary Web search engines and databases on health which is reported to have received glowing reviews from the press and university libraries. For additional information, consult Chapter III under Search Engine Databases and Newswires or the following Web site.

http://www.internets.com

Selected Popular Major Search Engines Directories and Indexes

Search engines not uncommonly are rated in terms of "popularity". A select list of 16 of the more popular Search Engines, Directories, and Indexes can be found in Table VII.

Table VII-Selected Major Popular Commercial Search Engines, Directories, Indexes and WebCrawlers

• Alta Vista	altavista.com
• AOL	aol.com
• Excite	excite.com
• Fast Search	alltheweb.com
• Google	google.com
• HotBot	hotbot.com
• Infoseek/Go	infoseek.go.com
• Librarian's Index	lii.org
• LookSmart	looksmart.com
• Lycos	lycos.com
• MSN	msn.com
• NBCi	ncbi.com
• Netscape	netscape.com
• Northern Light	northernlight.com
• WebCrawler	webcrawler.com
• Yahoo	yahoo.com

Each of the above is reviewed in terms of health information offered, in Chapter IV: Author's List of Selected Useful Search Tools and Web Sites. Brief highlights on each of these popular search tools are as follows.

Some of the history and interrelationships of these 16 selected popular search engines, directories, indexes, and webcrawlers may be helpful in understanding the Web and these search tools.

AltaVista began operations in December 1995 and is now part of CMGI. It is one of the largest search engines on the Web and uses directory listings from Open Directory and LookSmart.

AOL began operations in October 1999. Categories and web site information are obtained mostly from Open Directory, now part of Netscape. Crawler based results, as backup directory information, are obtained from Inktomi.

Excite began operations in late 1995 and purchased Magellan in July 1996 and WebCrawler in November 1996. Both acquisitions are run as separate services.

FastSearch was established July 1997 in Norway. A US subsidiary was opened in 1998. In early 1999, Fast Search entered into a partnership with Dell to build the world's largest search engine: one that would search all the Web. Recently Fast Search launched "all the Web, all the time" (http://www.alltheweb.com) toward this objective. This new Fast Search now claims to be the world's largest search engine with over 575 million URLs examining over 1.5 billion Web documents, the most of any search engine at the time this book was written. Fast Search now claims to handle some 12 million searches per day in a quick, easy and fast way with an average response time of well under a half second per search. It employs 32 individual language catalogues. Fast Search works closely with Lycos and LookSmart.

Google uses web link popularity to rank web sites and relevancy of information featured. It has a large index of the Web and provides results to Yahoo and Netscape.

HotBot began operations in May 1996. Results are obtained from DirectHit and Inktomi search engines while directory information is obtained from Open Directory. Lycos purchased HotBot in October 1998 and runs the company as a separate search tool and service.

Infoseek began operations in early 1995. Go was launched in January 1999.The combined company is Infoseek/Go which provides quality results thanks to its special search algorithm and an impressive human compiled directory of web sites and information.

The Librarian's Index to the Internet is a searchable, annotated subject directory of more than 7,000 Internet resources selected and evaluated by librarians for their usefulness to users of public libraries. It began in 1990 and was absorbed as the Berkley Public Library Index to the Internet in 1996. Afterward, a search engine was added along with subject index terms to which librarians add entries to this Index after careful evaluation.

LookSmart was launched in October 1996. It is a human compiled large directory of healthcare web sites/information. Also provides directory results to MSN, Excite and others.

Lycos began operations as a search engine in April 1999. It shifted to a directory model similar to Yahoo. Its main listings come from Open Directory and secondary results are obtained from Fast Search. HotBot was acquired in October 1998 but is run separately.

MSN is a LookSmart powered directory with secondary results coming from Inktomi.

NBCi began operations in November, 1999 as a combination of NBC and CNET's Search Tool, Snap.com, a human compiled directory of Web health information sites supplemented by search results from Inktomi. Snap.com was first launched in late 1997. One of Snap.com's reported goals, like Yahoo.com, is to categorize the entire Web.

Netscape uses information chiefly from Open Directory and Netscape's own "Smart Browsing" database. Google also provides information.

Northern Light began operation in August 1997 and features a large index of Web clustering documents by topic.

Open Directory was launched in June 1998 and uses volunteer editors to catalogue the Web. It was acquired by Netscape in November 1998. AltaVista, AOL, HotBot and Lycos all use Open Directory categories within their results pages for a licensing fee.

WebCrawler began operations in April, 1994 by the University of Washington. It features the smallest, useful index of any of the major commercial search engines and provides less overwhelming results in response to general searches. Subsequently it was purchased by Excite, which continues to run the business as an independent search tool.

Yahoo, launched in late 1994, is one of the Web's most popular search tools. It is reported to have one of the largest human compiled guide to the web health care information and supplements its results from Google. Yahoo is regarded as the oldest major directory.

The field of search engines, directories, and indexes and their interrelationships will continue to change rapidly. Interrelationships, similarities and differences should be considered in selecting any given search engine, directory, or index to obtain information. Results to any search may differ widely in terms of whether or not they are relevant, current, complete, or reliable. As a result, it is recommended that if one uses a popular, major commercial search engine, directory, or index to obtain information, one should do so using at least 3 or more different ones and compare and contrast results before reaching any conclusions with your physician or healthcare provider(s).

There are literally thousands of search tools available for obtaining health information. The exact number is in a state of flux because new ones are being created rapidly. Others are being merged and some are even going, or will be going out of business in the not too distant future for a number of reasons, mainly financial, even some of those reviewed in this book. All this could affect not only the existence of any given search tool, but also the quality of health information offered. Thus, the reader is cautioned to "adopt and stick with the best" and use ones that are likely to stay in business, maintaining their reputation and quality of health information provided and grow along with the Web healthcare information available.

Selected US Government Search Tools

Selected US Government Search Tools which may be regarded as reasonably current, evidence based, comprehensive and reliable for healthcare information are listed in Table VIII.

Table VIII-Selected Major US Government Search Tools

Search Tool Resource	Web Site
• Centers for Disease Control and Prevention	cdc.gov
• First Government	firstgov.gov
• Healthfinder	healthfinder.gov
• Medline	nlm.nih.gov/medline
• Medlineplus	nlm.nih.gov/medlineplus
• National Institutes of Health	nih.gov/health
• National Library of Medicine	nlm.nih.gov
• National Network of Libraries of Medicine	nnlm.nlm.nih.gov/psr
• PubMed	ncbi.nlm.nih.gov/PubMed

An outline of the information contained in each of the above web sites can be found in Chapter IV.

Of these, the Centers for Disease Control and Prevention, Healthfinder, Medlineplus and PubMed provide quick and easy access to a wealth of information on health and wellness and healthcare issues and topics, diseases and conditions, and treatment not only for the general public and patients but also for healthcare professionals alike. Detailed, more in depth information for patients, healthcare professionals and researchers may be obtained via Centers for Disease Control and Prevention, First Government, Medline, National Institutes of Health, National Library of Medicine and National Network of Libraries of Medicine.

Medical Colleges, Universities and Hospital Medical Centers

Medical Colleges, Universities and Hospital Medical Centers also provide current, evidence based, comprehensive and reliable information.

The Internet Medical School Directory (http://ds.dial.pipex.com/r.bowyer/med_sch.htm) contains a list of medical schools which provide easily accessible sources of healthcare information. Medical Schools sites listed are indexed alphabetically by country and by state in the United States. A number of these Medical College, Universities and Hospitals and their Web sites (i.e., Cornell, Duke, Emory, Harvard, Johns Hopkins, Mayo Clinic, Pittsburgh, Tufts, etc.) can be found in Chapter IV (Author's List) and Chapter VI Health Resources and Web Sites. The Association of American Medical Colleges Web site (http://www.aamc.org) also provides Web access to all Medical Colleges listed in their directory.

University affiliated hospital medical centers also may provide, current, reliable health, wellness and healthcare information. The Internet Hospital Directory (http://ds.dial.pipex,com/ r.bowyer/ hospital.htm) contains a list of hospitals accessible via the Web. Hospitals are listed alphabetically as well as by country, and state in the United States. You may click on to the site of your choice for health information available.

Further information on hospitals can be obtained via resources and Web sites provided in Chapter V, Health Categories, Diseases, Resources, and Web Sites.

Chapter IV

Author's List of Selected Useful Search Tools and Web Sites

This section contains an alphabetical list of 70 Search Tools and their corresponding Web sites, which have been researched by the author and considered to be useful. Basic health information on each is organized into categories to simplify and expedite searches. In the event that the information you are looking for is not available or is not sufficient, you can go to the search site provided within the search tool of your choice to obtain information on the topic in question.

Bear in mind that Search Tools described in this section of the book use different methods to search the Web and organize and categorize information collected. Thus, they may provide different results for any health topic searched. Not uncommonly, what you may or may not find via one search tool, you may be more pleased with on another. Therefore, it is prudent that you familiarize yourself with at least three or more search tools and compare and contrast results

For most healthcare information searches, the following 15 sites are regarded by the author as useful places to start your search:

• Commercial sites: Achoo, Google, Netscape and Yahoo

- Government sites: Healthfinder, National Institutes of Health, National Library of Medicine, Medlineplus and PubMed
- International sites: Health on the Net (Switzerland), Karolinska Institute (Sweden) and University of Hertfordshire (United Kingdom)
- University and Medical Center sites: Mayo Clinic Health Oasis, Intelihealth, and Harvard Medical Web

To start a search I tend to prefer: Google Web Directory, Fast Search, (All The Web), Harvard Medical Web, Healthfinder, Intelihealth, Mayo Clinic Health Oasis, Medlineplus, PubMed or Yahoo. However, depending on the health information needed, it may be more appropriate to revise the selection of starting Search Tools used. While you may start with one or more of the Search Tools suggested, in the long run, you need to select Search Tools that you find are most suitable for you own needs. Thus, your list of suitable search tools may turn out to be very much the same or different from the ones suggested.

Author's List of Selected Useful Search Tools, Web Sites

Search Tools

Achoo Gateway to Healthcare
Alta Vista: Health Web Directory
American Medical Association
American On Line Web Centers: Health
BioMedNet
Centers for Disease Control and Prevention
Doctor's Guide to the Internet
Dr. Koop.com
Drug Info Net
Duke University Healthy Devil Online

Excite Health
Fast Search (All The Web)
First Government
Google Web Directory: Health
Health Answers
Health Directory
Healthfinder
Health Gate
Health on the Net Foundation (Switzerland)
HotBot Directory: Health
Infoseek: Health and Wellness
Intelihealth
Karolinska Institutet (Sweden)
Librarian's Index to the Internet
Looksmart: Personal Health
Lycos Directory: Health
Magellan Health
Mayo Clinic Health Oasis
MD Consult
Med Explorer
Med Help International
Medical Matrix
Medicine Net.com
Medline (National Library of Medicine)
Medlineplus
Medscape
Med Web (Emory University Health Science)
MSN
National Cancer Institute
National Center for Complementary Alternative Medicine
National Center on Sleep Disorders
National Eye Institute

National Heart, Lung and Blood Institute
National Human Genome Research Institute
National Institute on Aging
National Institute on Alcohol Abuse and Alcoholism
National Institute of Allergy and Infectious Diseases
National Institute of Arthritis and Musculoskeletal
Diseases and Skin Diseases
National Institute of Child Health and Human Development
National Institute on Deafness and Other Communication Disorders
National Institute on Dental and Craniofacial Research
National Institute of Diabetes and Digestive and Kidney Diseases
National Institute on Drug Abuse
National Institute of Environmental Health Sciences
National Institutes of Health: Health Information
National Institute of Mental Health
National Institute of Neurological Disorders and Stroke
National Library of Medicine
National Network of Libraries of Medicine
NBCi.com:Health
Net Wellness
Netscape: Health
Northern Light Search
PubMed (National Library of Medicine)
Search Engine Databases and Newswires
University of Hertfordshire (United Kingdom)
WebCrawler Health
WebMD
Wellness Web
Yahoo Health

Achoo Gateway to Healthcare (Human Health and Disease Directory) http://www.achoo.com/directory/hhd/asp

Human Health and Disease Directory features sites on:
- Alternative medicine
- Dental health
- Diseases and conditions
- Drugs
- Exercise and fitness
- General health
- Human anatomy
- Laboratory and therapeutic procedures
- Medical ethics
- Medical sciences
- Mental health
- Nutrition
- Poisons
- Public and environmental health

Diseases and Conditions provides sites for information on:

- Bacterial and fungal diseases
- Blood and lympathic diseases
- Cancer
- Cardiovascular diseases
- Digestive system diseases
- Ear, nose and throat diseases
- Eye disease
- Female genital disease and pregnancy
- Immunological disease
- Injury, occupational disease
- Musculoskeletal diseases
- Neonatal diseases and abnormalities
- Nervous system disease
- Nutritional and metabolic diseases

- Parasitic diseases
- Respiratory tract diseases
- Skin and connective tissue diseases
- Symptoms and general pathology
- Urologic and male genital diseases
- Virus diseases

Additional information on any health topic of interest may be obtained by clicking on the Achoo Search sites for Medline, Merck Manual, the Internet, On Health Daily Briefings, or Mayo Clinic Health News.

Organizations and Sources provides information sites on

- Associations, Agencies and Organizations
- Computers and Medicine
- Conferences
- Databases and Directories
- Educational Institutions and Hospitals
- Electronic Journals and Periodicals
- Support Groups

Alta Vista: Health Web Directory
http:dir.altavista.com/top/health

Extensive healthweb directory. Categories of health information featured include:

- Alternative medicine
- Conditions and diseases
- Consumer support groups
- Dentistry
- Disabilities

- Emergency services
- Environmental health
- Fitness
- Health insurance
- Home health
- Life extension
- Medicine
- Mental health
- Nursing
- Nutrition
- Occupational health and safety
- Organizations
- Pharmacy/medications
- Professions
- Resources
- Search-health topics of interest
- Senses
- Services
- Substance abuse
- Weight loss

American Medical Association
http://www.ama-assn.org
http://ama-assn.org.org/consumer/gnrl.htm

Utilizes health web sites approved according to AMA guidelines for Medical and Health Information on the Internet (for guideline details, click on Web Guidelines or use direct web site as follows: http://www.ama-assn.org/about/guidelines.htm). The AMA Journals online you can click on directly include, among other:
- *Journal of the American Medical Association (JAMA)-*
- *Archives of Internal Medicine*

Consumer Health Information sites featured include:

- Antibiotic basics
- Blood transfusion
- Choosing your health plan
- Exercise benefits
- Fitness basics
- Healthy traveler
- Hospital finder
- Human atlas
- Laboratory tests
- Medical education
- Medical glossary
- Medical group practice finder
- Nutrition
- Person/family health history
- Physician finder
- Radiology tests
- Smoking cessation
- Tips from Dr. Wellbear
- Vitamins
- Your medical care

Information Centers sites include:

- Adolescent health
- Health insight
- HIV and AIDS
- Kid's health
- Migraine
- Women's health

Use AMA Search site to obtain additional information on health topics of interest.

America On Line Web Center: Health
http://www.aol.com/webcenters/health/home.adp

Click on Health to obtain information provided in the following sites:
Calculators and Quizzes

• Are You at Risk for HIV
• Are You Depressed
• Are You Fat
• Are You Getting Enough Sleep
• Are You too Stressed
• Do You Have Asthma
• Do You Smoke too Much
• *Health Information*
• *How Many Calories Do You Burn in a Day*
• *How Much Weight Can You Lose by Adding an Activity*
• Which Sports Burn the Most Calories

Conditions A to Z Search
Departments

• Babies and pregnancy
• Children's health
• Conditions and treatments
• Diet and nutrition
• Fitness and sports medicine
• Health and beauty
• Men's health
• Senior's health

- Tests and tools
- Women's health

Health News
Essentials:

- Body-mass calculator
- Calorie counter
- Drug directory
- Medical dictionary
- Medical test handbook
- Vitamin guide

Expert Advice
Search for available information on:

- Aging
- Alternative
- Child health
- Conditions and diseases
- Consumers support groups
- Dentistry
- Disabilities
- Education
- Environmental health
- Health insurance
- Healthcare industry
- Home health
- Men's health
- Nursing
- Nutrition
- Occupational health and safety

- Organizations
- Pharmacy
- Professions
- Public health and safety
- Publications
- Reproductive health
- Resources
- Senior health
- Senses
- Services
- Substance abuse
- Teen health
- Weight loss
- Women's health

BioMedNet
http://www.bmn.com

Collection of resources for biological medical researchers, physicians, and patients. Includes reliable databases, reviews news, links and journals. Biomedical databases include Medline and Swiss Prot. This site includes over 150 biomedical full text access journals and Medline. Reviews provide for a trial of the new customizable life science review source. WebLinks covers over 3,500 reviewed biomedical websites.

Centers for Disease Control and Prevention
http://www.cdc.gov
http://cdc.gov/health

Features information sites for:

- CDC Prevention Guidelines

- Data and statistics
- Health topics A to Z
- Hoaxes and rumors
- News
- Search topics of interest
- Traveler's health

Doctor's Guide to the Internet
http://www.pslgroup.com
http://www.pslgroup.com/docguide.htm
http://www.pslgroup.com/diabetes
http://www.pslgroup.com/mediation
http://www.pslgroup.com/menopause

Features the latest medical information A to Z: including conferences and news services updated daily. Search for the disease, condition, or health topic site of interest. Choose your favorite language, journals, or sites of interest.

Dr. Koop.com
http://www.dr.koop.com/health

Provides a medical encyclopedia and comprehensive, reliable information on disease and conditions A to Z, family health, health resources, mental health, nutrition, weight loss, drugs, health insurance and more. Web sites, reviews, and ratings also are provided.

Drug Info Net
http://www.druginfonet.com

Comprehensive resource of information on health and medication topics plus links to related sites on the web. Sites featured include:

- Ask the doctor
- Drug and disease information
- Frequently asked questions/answers
- Government sites
- Healthcare information
- Healthcare news
- Health organization sites
- Hospitals online
- Medical reference study
- Medical schools online
- Pharmaceutical manufacturer information
- Search for any drug or health topic of interest

Duke University Healthy Devil Online
http:healthydevil.stuaff.duke.edu

Features information sites on:

- Allergy and asthma
- Cancer
- Contraception
- Cold and flu
- Eating disorders
- Fitness
- General health and wellness
- Heart
- Irritable Bowel Syndrome
- Meningococcal disease
- Men's health
- Mental health
- Migraine and headaches
- Nutrition

- Pregnancy options
- Safe sex
- Sexually transmitted disease
- Stress management
- Substance abuse
- Tobacco
- Travel health
- Women's health

Excite Health
http://www.excite.com/health

Provided by WebMD. Health Directory and other sites featured include:

- Alternative medicine
- Ask the expert
- Diet and nutrition
- Disabilities
- Diseases and condition A to Z
- Drugs
- Eating right
- Exercise and fitness
- For professionals
- Insurance
- Mental health
- Miscellaneous
- Procedures
- Quick reference
- Sexual health
- Search for any health topic of interest
- Support groups
- Tools and calculator

Eating right site provides information on weight control, support, healthy heart quiz, expert advice and healthy cooking.

Exercise and fitness site includes how to get started, target heart rate and expert advice.

Quick reference site enables one to find information and resources on disease/medical condition and drugs/medications.

Fast Search (All The Web)
http:// www.alltheweb.com
http:// www.fastsearch.com

Regarded as the world's largest search engine reported to be capable of searching the entire Web. Contains 32 individual language catalogues.

Click on Help site to learn how to search for health, wellness and healthcare information using both Simple and Advanced Search options.

First Government
http://www.firstgov.gov
http://www.firstgov.gov/topics/healthy.html

Official website for searching the US Government resources. Provides current information about health, drugs, insurance and safety as well as medical references.

Featured links include Health, Insurance, Diseases.

Related links are provided for information on:

• Alcohol and drugs
• Alzheimer's Disease
• Asthma management
• Cancer
• Child health insurance
• Clinical practice guidelines

- Clinical trails
- Consumer health
- Drugs and medicines
- Health assessments
- Health promotion and disease prevention
- Healthcare for military
- Healthcare for veterans
- Healthy People By 2010
- Health research
- Heart disease prevention
- HIV and AIDS
- Insure Kids Now
- Medicare
- Medicaid
- Mental health
- Nursing homes
- Obesity
- Public health
- Quality of Healthcare Guide
- Smoke free kids
- Vaccination
- US Department of Health and Human Services
- Women's health

When you click on to the links above, you will leave this Web site and go to another Federal Government web site which provides the information sought.

Search Tips and Key Word Search For as well as a Search For sites are provided for you to obtain further information.

Google Web Directory: Health
http://google.com

http://www.directory.google.com/top/health

Categories of health information featured include:

- Aging
- Alternative medicine
- Child health
- Condition and diseases A to Z
- Consumer support groups
- Dentistry
- Disabilities
- Education
- Environmental health
- Fitness
- Health insurance
- Healthcare industry
- Home health
- Medicine
- Men's health
- Mental health
- Non-English sites
- Nursing
- Nutrition
- Occupational health and safety
- Organizations
- Pharmacy
- Professions
- Public health and safety
- Publications
- Reproductive health
- Resources
- Senior health

- Senses
- Services
- Substance abuse
- Teen health
- Weight loss
- Women's health

Conditions and Diseases categories include:

- Allergies
- Blood disorders
- Cancer
- Cardiovascular disorders
- Communication disorders
- Digestive disorders
- Ear, nose and throat disorders
- Endocrine disorder
- Eye disorders
- Gastrointestinal disorders
- Genetic disorders
- Immune disorders
- Infectious disease
- Mental health disorders
- Musculoskeletal disorders
- Neurological disorders
- Rare disorders
- Search conditions and diseases A to Z
- Sexually transmitted diseases
- Skin disorders
- Sleep disorders
- Urological disorders

Google Web Directory: Health, Medicine, Medical Specialities
http://www.directory.google.com/top.health/Medicine/Medical_Spec
ialities

Medical Specialties categories of information are:

- Aerospace medicine
- Allergist
- Anestesiology
- Behavorial medicine
- Cardiology
- Community health
- Critical care
- Dermatology
- Diving medicine
- Emergency medicine
- Endocrinology
- Epidemiology
- Family medicine
- Forensic science
- Gastroenterology
- Geriatrics
- Hematology
- Immunology
- Internal medicine
- Microbiology
- Multispeciality group
- Nephrology
- Neurology
- Nuclear medicine
- Ob-Gyn
- Occupational medicine

- Oncology
- Opthalmology
- Osteopathy
- Pain management
- Pathology
- Pediatrics
- Podiatry
- Psychiatry
- Pulmonary medicine
- Radiology
- Radiotherapy
- Rehabilitation medicine
- Rheumatology
- Rural health
- Sports medicine
- Surgery
- Toxicology
- Tropical health
- Wilderness medicine

Health Answers
http://www.healthanswers.com

Features sites on:

- Diseases and conditions A to Z
- Drug database
- Find it fast search
- Forums for chat and discussion
- Healthcenters/topics A to Z
- Health tools
    - Body mass calculator

• Heart disease risk factors
• Media news center
• Medical encyclopedia
• Newsletter (free)
• Search site for health topics
  • of interest

      • Calorie burner
      • Heart rate calculator

Subscribes to the HON code of principles of Health on the Net Foundation.

Health Directory
http://www.healthdirectory.com

A strategic partnership and licensing agreement was formed in October 2000 with Medidas, Korea's leading provider of medical information since 1994.

Health Directory features click on sites for:

• Condition Center
• Dictionary
• Medical libraries
• Medical news
• Medical societies
• Resource center
• Search engine

Dictionary is a searchable tool of medical specialties.

Condition Center reports on various medical topics which are written and updated by experienced medical writers and reviewed and edited by in house editors and a board of physicians at Harvard Medical School and Massachusetts General Hospital.

Medical Libraries provides links to medical libraries, news outlets, and Internet Search Engines that provide current health and medical information.

Medical news is by top health and news outlets.

Medical societies and Resources provide links to medical societies and professional organizations and more.

Search Engine site enables one to search for the most relevant and useful health and medical web sites on the Internet.

Healthfinder
http://www.healthfinder.gov

U.S. Department of Health and Human Services Web site for comprehensive, health, wellness and healthcare information. Site may assist you to stay healthier, understand diagnoses, disease, conditions, explore treatment options, find support, and generally become more informed about health and medical topics. Use Healthfinder's 9 point checklist to help you decide if any health Web site information is reasonably reliable.

Health Topics featured on Healthfinder include:

• Adults
• AIDS
• Alternative medicine
• Cancer
• Children
• Databases
• Diabetes
• Families

- Food safety
- Foreign language resources
- Government health news
- Health media online
- Health information online
- Health information toll free
- Infants
- Journals
- Libraries
- Links
- Medical dictionaries
- Men's and women's health
- Minority health
- Prevention and self care
- Professionals
- Quality care choices
- Medicare
- Search engines and health sites
- Seniors
- Support and self help
- Teens
- Tobacco

For a directory of advocacy groups or professional organizations, click on "Professionals" site under health topics.

You may use the Healthfinder search site to obtain information on health topics of interest.

HealthGate
http://www.healthgate.com

An important online source for health, wellness and biomedical information. HealthGate allows visitors to search Medline, CancerLit and the MDX Family Health Library at no charge. Medical research tool for consumers, patients, physicians and professionals. Sites featured include:

- Aging and health
- Alternative health
- Conditions and concerns
- Food and nutrition
- Health calculators
- Health news
- Medical dictionary
- Medications
- Men's health
- Mental health
- Search site
- Sexuality and health
- Sports and fitness
- Teen's/kid's health
- Travel and health
- Weekly briefings

Subscribes to the HON Code of Conduct of the Health on the Net Foundation.

Health on the Net Foundation (Switzerland)
http://www.hon.ch

Key international search engine for healthcare information, headquartered in Geneva, Switzerland. Its Medhunt search engine ranks various Web health sites by a scoring system and allows for the search of health information to be narrowed quickly and easily. Direct access to Medline, Medhunt, MeSH as well as other databases is provided.

Honselect combines five information types: 1) MeSH terms, 2) authoritative scientific articles, 3) healthline news, 4) Web sites, and 5) multimedia into one service and expedites your search for health care information. Browse over 30,000 MeSH terms or select a subject from popular categories. Or you may enter a specific health topic and search, or you may choose from an A to Z list of healthcare topics by clicking on "Favorites" which includes an alphabetical selection of the most searched health topics with HON services.

Other HON topics featured include:

- Support communities: list, frequently asked questions and answers, and a wide range of information
- Media gallery: searchable database of medical images and movies from various sources.
- HON projects: efforts to build and improve health information on the Internet with the HON Code of Conduct.
- Conferences and events: healthcare conferences past, present and upcoming
- HON library: papers from conferences and other medical sources
- Surveys: results of surveys on Internet usage for healthcare purposes
- Daily healthcare news

HotBot Directory: Health
http://www.dir.hotbot.lycos.com/health

Thousands of pages on all aspects of health brought to you by WebMD. Sites featured include:

- Aging
- Alternative medicine

- Child health
- Conditions and diseases A to Z
- Consumer Support Groups
- Dentistry
- Disabilities
- Education
- Environmental health
- Fitness
- Health insurance
- Healthcare industry
- Home health
- Hospitals
- Medicine
- Men's health
- Mental health
- Nursing
- Nutrition
- Occupational health and safety
- Organizations
- Pharmacy/medications
- Professions
- Public health and safety
- Publications
- Reproductive health
- Resources
- Searchable databases
- Senior health
- Senses
- Services
- Substance abuse
- Teen health
- Weight loss

• Women's health

Featured in Lycos Health Network are:

• Health articles A to Z: topics picked by WebMD team of medical researchers on illnesses, conditions and concerns
• Health encyclopedia: health from A to Z
• Health experts: opinions and knowledge on topics like diet, emotional wellness, men's health and parenting
• Health news headlines: comprehensive collections of current health-related news headlines

Infoseek: Health and Wellness
http://www.infoseek.com
http://www.go.com/WebDir/health
http://www.infoseek.go.com/center/health

Features sites including:

• Disease and condition A to Z
• Family health
• Fitness
• Health and wellness
• Nutrition
• Prevention center
• Preventionaire
• Tackling tobacco
• Weight loss
• Health news
• Health resources
• Healthtopics
• Medical reference

- Medications-drug checker
- Medical encyclopedia
- Mental health

Medical reference topics featured include:

- American Heart Association
- Blood donation
- Body fat composition
- Care giving
- Centers for Disease Control
- Clinical trials
- Community health issues
- CPR
- First aid
- Genetic counseling
- Genetic engineering
- Health and fitness
- Healthcare decision
- Health chat
- Health conferences
- Health discussion groups
- Health hotlines
- Health media
- Health tools
- Heimlich maneuver
- History of medicine
- Human anatomy
- Longevity
- Medical associations
- Medical dictionaries
- Medical encyclopedias

- Medical journals
- Medical libraries
- Medical malpractice
- Medical museums
- Medical news
- Mortality
- National Institutes of Health
- Nobel Prize
- Non-toxic living
- Office US Surgeon General
- Online health programs
- Patient's rights
- Personal health test
- Physician's assistants
- Physician Desk Reference
- Placebo effect
- Poison control centers
- Preventive medicine
- Public health
- Self exams
- Surgery webcasts
- Travel health
- Universal health care
- Wellness
- Wound care

Search Dr. Koop and Drug checker sites also are available. Ratings of health web sites reviewed are provided.

Intelihealth
http://www.intelihealth.com

Features Harvard Medical School's Consumer health Information site for current information.

Intelihealth Home Site provides a collection of consumer health information sites. Featured sites include:

- Allergy
- Arthritis
- Asthma
- Babies
- Cancer
- Care givers
- Chats
- Children's health
- Diabetes
- Digestive disorders
- Diseases and conditions A to Z
- Drug search
- Drug resource center
- Fitness
- Headache
- Health A-Z
- Heart
- HIV and AIDS
- Managed health
- Medical dictionary
- Men's health
- Mental health
- Nutrition
- Pregnancy
- Resources
- Search Intelihealth
- Sexual and reproductive health

- Sports medicine
- Vitamins
- Weight management
- Women's health

Karolinska Institutet (Sweden)
http://www.mic.ki.se/diseases/index.html

Leading international health information web site located in Stockholm, Sweden. Provides key international health information and sites for:

- Biomedical links
- Diseases, disorders and related topics. MeSH classified resources on the Internet for the general public, patients, healthcare professionals and researchers. You may click on to an alphabetical list of diseases A to Z and then click on a selected entry to go to relevant MeSH page(s) and information on that disease.
- Electronic journals
- Medline and databases
- Subject information on:
    - Ask the Doctor and Second Opinion Services
    - Anesthesia and analgesia
    - Bacterial infections and mycoses
    - Bioethics
    - Biological sciences
    - Behavior and mental disorders
    - Dentistry
    - Diagnosis
    - Digestive system diseases
    - Disorders of environmental origin
    - Endocrine diseases

- Eye disease
- Female genital diseases and pregnancy complications
- Hemic (blood) and lymphatic diseases
- Immunologic disease
- Medical images
- Medical news
- Musculoskeletal disease
- Neonatal disease and abnormalities
- Neoplasms
- Nervous system disease
- Nutritional and metaboloic disease
- Otorhinolayringological disease (ear, nose, throat)
- Parasitic disease
- Pathological conditions, signs and symptoms
- Respiratory disease
- Skin and connective tissue disease
- Stomatognathic disease (mouth, jaw)
- Surgical procedures, operative dentistry
- Therapeutics/drugs
- Urologic and male genital disease
- Virus disease

Librarians' Index To The Internet
http://www.lii.org

A librarian selected and annotated index to health on the Internet.
Click on Health and go to Health and Medicine General Resources.
Sites featured are:

- Acupuncture
- Aged care
- Alternative medicine

- Anatomy
- Blood
- Brain
- Breast feeding
- Childbirth
- Children's health
- Chinese medicine
- Chiropractic
- Clinical trials
- Counseling
- Death
- Dentistry
- Dermatology
- Disabilities
- Diseases and conditions
- Drugs
- Ear
- Emergency medicine
- Epidemiology
- Ergonomics
- Euthanasia
- Exercise
- Eye
- Genetics
- Grief
- Heart
- History
- Hospices
- Hospitals
- Infants (premature)
- Insurance
- Long term care

- Medical records
- Medicaid and Medicare
- Medicinal plants
- Meditation
- Medline
- Men's health
- Mental health
- Midwives
- Muscles
- Nursing
- Nutrition
- Orthopedics
- Pediatrics
- Physicians
- Physiology
- Pregnancy
- Psychology
- Radiation
- Reproduction
- Senses
- Sleep
- Surgery
- Toxicology
- Transplants
- Vaccines
- Veterinary medicine
- Virology
- Women's health

Other sites you may click on are: Dictionaires, Food, Medicine, Organizations, Recreation, Reference Desk and Searching the Internet/Web.

Look Smart: Health
http://www.looksmart.com/health

Click on Health under the heading Personal. Sites featured include:

• Guides and directories
• Conditions/illnesses A to Z
• Diet and nutrition
• Drugs and medicine
• Family and community
• Fitness and exercise
• Hospitals and services
• Health calculators
• Health newsgroups
• Life and health insurance
• Medical guides
• Medical tips
• Natural therapies
• Public health
• Reference news
• Search for health topics of interest
• Sexual health
• Weight management

Lycos Directory: Health
http:/ www.dir.lycos.com/health

Information is provided in conjunction with WebMD on:

• Alternative medicine
• Aging
• Animals

- Beauty
- Child health
- Condition and diseases A to Z
- Consumer support groups
- Dentistry
- Disabilities
- Education
- Employment
- Environmental health
- Fitness
- Health articles A to Z
- Health encyclopedia
- Health experts
- Health insurance
- Health news
- Healthcare industry
- Home health
- Medicine
- Mental health
- Nursing
- Nutrition
- Occupational health and safety
- Organizations
- Pharmacy
- Products and shopping
- Professions
- Public health and safety
- Publications
- Reproductive health
- Resources
- Searchable databases
- Senior health

- Senses
- Services
- Substance abuse
- Teen health
- Weight loss
- Women's health
- WebMD Wellness Center
- Search for health topics of interest

Magellan: Health
http://www.magellan.excite.com/health

Click on Health. Sites featured include:

- Alternative medicine
- Diet and nutrition
- Disabilities
- Diseases and conditions
- Drugs
- Exercise and fitness
- Family health
- For professionals
- Insurance
- Mental health
- Miscellaneous
- More sites: dictionaries, etc.
- Procedures
- Quick reference
- Recommended health and wellness
- Search for any health topic of interest
- Sexual health
- Support groups

• Tools and calculators

Mayo Clinic Health Oasis
http://www.mayohealth.org

A reliable web site for health and wellness information by the renowned Mayo Clinic. The breadth and depth of the Mayo Clinic's expertise enables them to provide current health information on a variety of topics and gives you access to the experience and knowledge of over 1,000 dedicated physicians and scientists. Centers and sites for health information featured include:

• Ask Mayo any question
• Allergy and asthma
• Arthritis
• Alzheimer's disease
• Cancer
• Children's health
• Digestive disorders
• Diseases and conditions A to Z
• Glossary of terms A to Z
• Headline news
• Health topics A to Z
• Heart disease
• Library
• Medicine
• Men's health
• Nutrition
• Search for drug information by name
• Search for health topics of interest
• Secrets of longevity
• Women's health

This site provides you with easy-to-read, relevant information for a healthier life, explanations on how to treat common and uncommon illnesses, as well as information on disease prevention.

Mayo Health Oasis subscribes to the HON Code of Conduct of the Health on the Net Foundation.

MD Consult
http://www.mdconsult.com

Provides quality patient oriented medical information for patients, families and health care professionals. Information and services are available for over 50 medical topics. MD Consult was founded by leading medical publishers, licensed by more than half of U.S. academic medical centers and used by physicians in over 70 countries. It employs reliable clinical content from over 50 sources. Features health information on:

- Answers to Medical Questions: via a number of outstanding medical texts online. Search the entire collection.
- Journal Search: retrieve the complete text of articles from medical journals and *Clinics of North America* online. Also, search Medline plus other key databases simultaneously.
- Practice Guidelines: easy to use guides to accepted practice. Hundreds of peer-reviewed clinical practice guidelines contributed by a number of medical societies and government agencies.
- Patient Education: patient education handouts on diseases and treatments with special instructions.
- Drug Information: updated prescribing information on thousands of medications
- Today in Medicine: latest developments in medicine. Reviews of new developments from major journals, government agencies and medical conferences providing concise clinical summaries and links to related information.

- What Patients Are Reading: reviews popular press information each week describing what patients are reading. Provides full text peer reviewed material on each topic.
- In This Week's Journal: contents of five key journals are presented each week in an easy-to-scan format including concise article summaries.
- Clinical Topic Tour: lets you explore current thought and accepted wisdom on consequential topics in medicine on a weekly basis.
- Drug Updates: FDA drug approvals and other current pharmaceutical information.

Med Explorer
http://www.medexplorer.com

Health and Medical Information Center site features:

- Allied health: occupational therapy, physical therapy, etc
- Alternative medicine: complementary medicine, associations
- Computers/software: education, fitness, health, safety, hearing impairment, imaging
- Community health: extended care, home health, long term care, medical clinics
- Conferences: posting of health and medical newsgroups
- Death and dying: palliative care, suicide, pro life resources
- Dentistry: cosmetic dentistry and dental alloys, anesthetics, centers, laboratories and implants,
- Diseases and disorders: search A to Z
- Education: community, conferences, continuing education
- Emergency services: aeromedical, disaster, emergency and medical
- Health exam: nutrition database, health news, Medline, BMI calculator
- Health insurance: insurance, claims, managed care, outpatient, prescription drug coverage

- Health nutrition: fitness, men's health, nutrition, parenting, family health
- Health safety: fire prevention and safety, hygiene, infection control, injury prevention, occupational health
- Hospitals: cardiac, cardiovascular, catholic, children's, clinics, emergency care, and more
- Laboratories: genetic testing, molecular oncology, resources
- Medical imaging: full service radiology, interventional therapy, radiology, resources
- Mental health: counseling, depression, eating disorders, education, hypnosis, journals, and more
- Miscellaneous: medical travel, parenting, family health
- Medexploring: objective web site reviews, health news
- Newsgroups: over 250 searchable health and medical newsgroups
- Nutrition database: for nutrition facts
- Pharmaceutical: drugs
- Research: diseases, and conditions A to Z
- Specialty medicine: disease and conditions A to Z
- Search: information of interest
- Vision: vision disorders

Med Help International
http://www.medhelp.org/home.htm

Dedicated to helping patients find current quality medical information throughout the world. Their Virtual Medical Center for Patients is a collection of information and professional medical support from the top medical organizations and experts worldwide comprised of:
- Comprehensive Consumer Health Information Library utilizing the Med Help Search Engine
- Questions and Answer Specialty Forums giving patients direct access to leading physicians and healthcare professionals

- Patient Network
- Daily Medical and Health News

Sites featured include:
- Ask the Doctor

  - Addiction
  - Child Behavorial Health
  - Dermatology
  - Gastroenterology
  - Heart
  - Hepatitis
  - Incontinence
  - Liver Diseases
  - Mental Health
  - Neurology
  - Neurosurgery
  - Transplants
  - Urologic Cancer

- Links
  - News
  - Patient Network
  - Search: Med Help Search Engine

Subscribes to the HON Code of Conduct of the Health On the Net Foundation and follows the AMA Code of Ethics in the best interests of the patient.

Medical Matrix
http://www.medicalmatrix.org

Directory of medical sites useful to both patients and health care practitioners. Provides links to quality sources listed by subject which have been reviewed by the Internet Working Group of the American Medical Association. Site provided to search for information on health topics of interest.

MedicineNet
http://www.medicinenet.com

Physician produced health, wellness and other medical information. Features sites for:

• Diseases and condition A-Z
• Doctors' views library
• First aid
• Health facts library
• Healthy living
• Medical links
• Medical dictionary
• Medications
• Procedures and tests
• Poison control
• Search for health topics of interest

Medline (National Library of Medicine)
http://www.nlm.nih.gov/medline

Medline is the National Library of Medicine's online database that contains more than 10 million references to journal articles in the health sciences. PubMed and Internet Grateful Med are two free systems to search Medline. Direct free access to Medline is also available via other search tools such as Health on the Net Foundation (http://www.hon.ch).

Medlineplus (National Library of Medicine)
http://www.nlm.nih.gov/medlineplus

Information on thousands of diseases, conditions, and wellness issues. Choose a topic by letter from A to Z from list of all topics or choose a tropic by category provided and search for desired information.

Sites provided for information on databases, dictionaries, doctors and dentists, drugs, hospitals, organizations, Medline, publications, and news, and Search Medlineplus.

Medscape
http://www.medscape.com

Designed for healthcare professionals and consumers. Offering one of the largest collection of free full-text and peer reviewed articles, medical news, Medline, and interactive quizzes. Updated daily. Databases offered for searches include:

- Aidsline
- Bookstore
- Clinical content
- Medical dictionary
- Medical images

- Medication information
- Medline
- News
- Patient information

Select one of the above databases above and enter a search term/topic to search for information of interest.

Other sites featured include:

- CBS Health Watch for Consumers
- Clinical management
- Conference schedules
- Conference summaries
- Exam room
- In focus health topics
- Journal room
- Library
- Managed care
- Multi specialty links
- Nurses
- Patient resources
- Pharmacists
- Practice guidelines
- Search for a physician
- Specialty spotlight
- Today on Medscape
- Today's health headlines
- Treatment updates

MedWeb (Emory University Health Sciences)
http://www.medweb.emory.edu/edu/medweb

MedWeb is a catalog of health related web sites maintained by the Emory Health Sciences Center Library, Emory University School of Medicine. Browse by subject or search for any health topic of interest A to Z.

MSN
http://www.msn.com
http://www.health.msn.com

MSN provides health, wellness and healthcare information in conjunction with WebMD. Click on Health. Sites featured include:

- Ask our experts
- Complementary medicine
- Daily chat schedule
- Diet and nutrition
- Drug reference
- Emotional wellness
- Fitness
- Focus on health
    - men
    - parenting
    - seniors
    - women
- Health and Women Central
- Health mall
- Health news
- Health professionals
- Health topic features
- Illnesses and conditions
- Insurance and legal matters
- Medical encyclopedia
- Online health communities
- Quick links
- Reference Library
- Relationships and sexuality
- Search for health
    - information of interest
- Self care advisor
- Today on health
- Try this

• WebMD Live Calendar

National Cancer Institute
http://www.nci.nih.gov

Provides cancer information, types of cancer, treatments, clinical trials, risk factors, publications and reports, statistics, health disparities, and advocacy groups, as well as 1-800-4-CANCER number for the latest, most accurate cancer information. Use NCI Search site for information on cancer topics of interest.

National Center for Complementary Alternative Medicine
http://www.nccam.nih.gov

As a leading Federal effort in the field, NCCAM conducts and supports basic and applied research and training and disseminates information on complementary and alternative medicine to practitioners and the public. Users are cautioned not to use the therapies described without the consultation of a licensed health provider. Inclusion of a treatment or resource on the Web site does not imply endorsement by NCCAM, the NIH, or the Department of Health and Human Services. A warning and disclaimer is provided regarding information made available.

Features sites for:

• Classification of CAM activities*
• Clearinghouse information **
• Clinical trials opportunities
• Consensus reports
• Databases
• Fact sheets
• For consumers and practitioners

- For investigators
- Frequently asked questions and answers
- News
- Research information
- Search for CAM topics of interest
- What's new

*Categorization scheme developed by an ad hoc advisory panel to the NCCAM and further refined by the Workshop on Alternative Medicine

**Disseminates information to healthcare professionals, media and the public to promote complementary alternative medicine awareness, education and research.

National Center on Sleep Disorders
http://www.nhlbi.nih.gov/about/ncsdr/index.htm

National Center on Sleep disorders is organizationally part of the National Health, Lung and Blood Institute. Click on National Center on Sleep Disorders Research. Provides information and resources on an array of sleep disorders for patients, professionals and the public.

National Eye Institute
http://www.nei.nih.gov

Leading U.S. Government effort regarding research, diagnosis, and treatment of eye disorders. Supports the vast majority of the vision research conducted in the United States at approximately 250 medical centers, hospital, universities, and other institutions, as well as its own facilities in Bethesda, Maryland, to combat the myriad of eye disorders affecting millions of people worldwide. Provides information sites on a variety of eye disorders including:

- Cataracts
- Corneal transplants
- Diabetic retinopathy
- Glaucoma
- Macular degeneration
- Retinal detachment
- Refractive surgery
- Vision problems and other

Use NEI search site to obtain further information on eye disorders and topics of interest.

National Heart, Lung and Blood Institute
http://www.nhlbi.nih.gov

For cardiovascular information click on Health Information and then Cardiovascular Information. Topics featured for patients and/or professionals include:

- Cholesterol
- Heart attack information
- High blood pressure
- Latino cardiovascular health resources
- Obesity
- Other cardiovascular information
- Search topics of interest

Lung Information: click on Health Information and then Lung Information which features sites for patients and/or professionals:

- Asthma
- Emphysema

- List of publications
- Lung cancer
- Other lung information
- Search for further information
    - on lung and its disorders

Blood Diseases and Resources: click on Health Information and then Blood Diseases and Resources for information on:

- Additional blood resources
- Blood transfusion safety
- Links to other blood disease sites
- List of publications
- NCI for cancers of the blood
- Other blood information on:
    - Check your blood IQ
    - Hemophilia
    - Thrombocytopenia purpura
    - Raynaud's phenomenon
- Search for information on blood topics of interest
- Sickle cell disease

Heart, lung and blood information may also be accessed directly via the following web sites:
- http://www.nhlbi.nih.gov/health/public/heart/index.htm
- http://www.nhlbi.nih.gov/health/prof/heart/index.htm
- http://www.nhlbi.nih.gov/health/public/lung/index.htm
- http://www.nhlbi.nih.gov/health/prof/lung/index.htm
- http://www.nhlbi.nih.gov/health/public/blood/index.htm

National Human Genome Research Institute
http://www.nhgri.nih.gov.index.html

Primary Federal effort regarding medical genetics. Features information on:

• Center for Inherited Disease Research
• Ethical, legal and social implication
• Genomic and genetic resources
• Glossary of genetic terms
• Intramural research
• News
• Policy and public affairs
• Search for further information on
  medical genetics topics of interest

National Institute on Aging
http://www.nih.gov/nia

Leading Federal effort regarding aging and health. Provides sites for:

• Health information
• National Advisory Council on Aging
• News and events
• Research programs
• Search for information on aging topics of interest

National Institute on Alcohol Abuse and Alcoholism
http://www.niaa.nih.gov

Leading U.S. Government effort regarding alcohol abuse and alcoholism. Features sites for information on:

• Conferences and events
• Databases

- ETOH (ethanol) database: alcohol and alcohol problems science database
- Clinical trials database
- National Library of Medicine Databases and Electronic Sources: access to a variety of resources related to biomedical and health sciences including:
  - Medline: premier database covering the fields of medicine, nursing, dentistry, the health care system, and the preclinical sciences and,
  - Medlineplus: consumer health information network on diseases, conditions and wellness issues
- Frequently asked questions and answers
- Other resources: links to referral information on related organizations and associations sites
- Press releases and other publications
- Research programs

National Institute of Allergy and Infectious Diseases
http://www.niaid.nih.gov

Leading U.S. Government effort on allergy and infectious diseases. Features information sites on:

- Activities
- Allergies
- Infectious disease
- Publications
- Research
- Search for information on
  allergy or infectious disease topics of interest
- Shingles prevention

National Institute of Arthritis and Musculoskeletal and Skin Diseases
http://www.nih.gov/niams
http://www.nih.gov/niams/healthinfo.gov
http://www.nih.gov/niams/healthinfo.gov

Provides information on many forms of arthritis and diseases of the musculoskeletal system and skin. The Institute also conducts and supports basic research on the normal structure and function of joints, muscles, bones and skin. Addresses the fields of rheumatology, orthopedics, dermatology, metabolic bone diseases, heritable disorders of bone and cartilage, inherited and inflammatory muscle disease, and sports and rehabilitation medicine. Features information sites on:

- Additional sources of information: links to other biomedical resources on the internet
- Clinical studies: information on clinical research and protocols, patient enrollment and results of clinical trials
- Health information: brochures, fact sheets, health statistics, how to order information and resources
- News and events: agendas for upcoming meetings, announcements, calendar of events and news releases
- Reports: publications and contributions to NIH reports
- Search site: for further information on any arthritis, musculoskeletal or skin disease topic of interest
- Scientific resources: bibliographies, consensus conference reports and scientific research databases

National Institute of Child Health and Human Development
http://www.nichd.nih.gov

Comprehensive U.S. government effort concerning child health and human development.

Features information sites on:

- Epidemiology: Division of Epidemiology, Statistics, and Prevention Research
- Health information and media: resources for consumer health information, publications, information on milk matters and news
- Intramural research: research activities of the Institute
- News and events: news releases, conferences, new policies and items new to the site
- Strategic planning: fetal tissue research, health disparities strategic plan and teaching children to read
- Research resources: information and materials for use by researchers
- Search site: for information on any child health and human development topic of interest

National Institute on Deafness and Other Communication Disorders
http://www.nih.gov/nidcd

Provides information on and supports human communication and deafness research. Features sites on:

- Frequently asked questions and answers
- Health information regarding:
    - Clinical trials
    - Directory of organizations
    - Hearing and balance
    - Kids and teachers
    - Parent's considerations
    - Publications
    - Smell and taste
    - Voice, speech and language
- Intramural research

- Basic research program
- Clinical research program
- Intramural scientists
- Research opportunities
- News and events
  - Research updates
  - Meetings
- Search for additional information on communication and deafness
- Strategic planning
  - National strategic research plan
  - Single and multiple project reports

National Institute of Dental and Craniofacial Research
http://www.nidcr.nih.gov/cranio/disease/ac.html
http://www.nidcr.nih.gov/news/publica.htm

Leading U.S. Government effort on dental and craniofacial disorders research. Features information sites on:

- About faces/craniofacial knowledge
- Healthcare and patient information
- Insights on human health
- News and health
- On oral health, Surgeon General's Report
- Research
- Resource linkages
- Search for additional information on
  dental and craniofacial disorders
- Sjogren's Syndrome clinic
- Spectrum Series
- Science workshop reports
- Vision 2020: NIH heads foresee the future

National Institute of Diabetes and Digestive and Kidney Diseases
http://www.niddk.nih.gov

Leading U.S. Government effort concerning diabetes, digestive and kidney disease. Comprehensive patient/consumer information provided via following featured sites:

- Clinical trials
- Diabetes education program
- Frequently asked questions and answers
- Health education programs
- Health information A to Z list of topics
    and other resources to choose from
- Laboratories/scientific databases
    and resources
- Minority health disparities
- National information
  clearinghouses/reports
- News briefs and releases
- Research efforts
- Search for additional information
    on diabetes, digestive disorders and
    kidney diseases
- Strategic plans

National Institute on Drug Abuse
http://www.nida.nih.gov

Premier Federal effort providing comprehensive patient information on drug abuse. Information sites featured include:

- Drug abuse information

- International information
- Legislation
- News releases
- Organizations
- Other links
- Publications
- Quick search site for drug
    abuse topics of interest
- Research
- Scientific meetings and summaries
- What's new

Other sites provide information on:

- Clubdrugs.org: information about club drugs
- Drug Abuse and Addiction Research: Sixth Triennial Report to Congress on drug use and drug use research
- 5 year strategic plan
- Monitoring the Future Study: tracks alcohol and drug use by students in the 8th, 10th and 12th grades
- NIDA Notes: bimonthly newsletter covering substance abuse treatment and prevention, research, epidemiology, neuroscience, behavioral research, health services research, and AIDS
- Steroid abuse.org: for information about anabolic steroid abuse
- Tobacco use: transdisciplinary tobacco use research centers web site

National Institute of Environmental Health Sciences
http://www.niehs.nih.gov

Comprehensive information on environmental related disease. Featured sites include:

- Carcinogens
- Community outreach and contacts
- Environmental genome project
- Facts about environment-related
    Diseases and health risks
- Journals and electronic data service
- Kid's page
- Library
- National toxicology program
- News and events
- Scientific research
- Strategic plan
- Web search site for additional information

National Institutes of Health: Health Information
http://www.nih.gov/health

Three helpful ways of obtaining useful information from the World Wide Web are suggested, namely:

- NIH Health Information Index A to Z Subject Guide: provides direct links to a specific NIH Institute or Center that supports research and provides information related to the health topic of interest.
- Medlineplus: developed by medical reference librarians for the National Library of Medicine. Enables one to obtain reliable health information not only from NIH but also from other institutions across the United States.
- Clinical trials.gov: consumer friendly database of information on federal and private clinical trials involving patients and others at thousands of locations nationwide.

National Institute of Mental Health

http://www.nimh.nih.gov

Chief Federal effort regarding mental health. Features information sites on:

- Anxiety disorders
- Children and violence
- Clinical trials
- Conferences and workshops summaries
- Depressive disorders
- For practitioners
- For the public
- For researchers
- Highlights
- Material in Spanish
- Mental health Surgeon General's Report
- News and events
- Online ordering
- Publications
- Outreach and educational program
- Public alerts
- Search for mental health topics of interest
- Sequenced treatment alternatives to relieve depression
- Translating behavioral science into action
- What's new

National Institute of Neurological Disorders and Stroke
http://www.ninds.nih.gov

Central U.S. Government effort regarding neurological disorders and stroke. Features sites on:

- Disorder quick links
- Establishment of stroke centers to reduce deaths and disabilities
- Laboratories at NINDS
- Neurological disorders
- News and events
- Pediatric stroke
- Search for additional information on neurological disorders and stroke

National Library of Medicine (NLM)
http://www.nlm.nih.gov

Worlds largest medical library and creator of Medline. Provides detailed current information on:

- Clinical trials.gov: information for patients about clinical research studies
- General information: frequently asked questions and answers
- Go to Medlineplus: health information selected for you by NLM
- Health information: Medline, Medlineplus and other resources
- Library services: catalog, databases, publications
- News and noteworthy: news, hot topics
- Search NLM web site: health topics of interest
  - Databases
  - Dictionaries
  - Doctors/dentists
  - Drug information
  - Hospitals
  - Libraries
  - Medical encyclopedia
  - Medline
  - Medlineplus

• Publications and news

User will find information on thousands of diseases, conditions and wellness issues. Topics may be searched by letter or chosen from a list of topics or by category.

National Network of Libraries of Medicine
http://www.nnlm.nlm.nih.gov/psr

Information for U.S. health professionals, patients and the general public designed to advance the progress of medicine and improve the public health. Program is coordinated by the National Library of Medicine via a nationwide network of health science libraries and information centers under contract with the Pacific Southwest Regional Library (PSRL) based at the Louise M. Darling Biomedical Library at the University of California at Los Angeles (UCLA).

NNLM recommends the following search tools and web sites useful for consumer health information:

• Medlineplus   http://www.nlm.nih.gov/medlinplus
Consumer health information. Utilizes a selective list of authoritative health information sources from the National Institutes of Health and other organizations to provide consumer health information on:
  • Clearinghouses: organizations that will send health literature to your home
  • Databases: articles and information from other organizations
  • Dictionaries: definitions of medical terms
  • Doctors and dentists: finding a doctor, dentist or other health professional
  • Health Topics: links to health information from NIH and other sources
  • Hospitals: finding a hospital or other health facility

- Libraries: find a nearby library for health consumers
- Publications and news: textbooks, newsletters and health news sources
- Medline http://www.nlm.nih.gov/medline
Online database with more than 10 million references to journal articles in the health sciences. PubMed and Internet Grateful Med are two free systems to search Medline.
- Healthfinder http://www.healthfinder.gov
Consumer health and human services information
- Center for Disease Control and Prevention http://www.cdc.gov
Answers about immunizations, health and quality of life by preventing and controlling disease, injury and disability
- Shape Up America http://www.shapeup.org
National initiative to promote weight control and increased physical activity
- National Women's Health Information Center http://www.woman.gov
Vast array of Federal and other women's health information resources
- Kid'sHealth.org http://www.kidshealth.org
Provides information on infections, behavior and emotions, food and fitness and growing up healthy.

NBCi.com: Health
http://www.nbci.com/directory/health

In Health information sites featured include:

- Alternative medicine
- Care providers
- Child and youth
- Dental
- Drugs and medications A to Z
- Fitness

- Medical conditions A to Z
- Men's
- Mental
- News
- Nutrition
- Public
- Senior
- Sexual
- Travel
- Weight loss
- Woman's

Features the following Medical Conditions sites:

- Birth defects
- Blood and circulatory
- Bone and skeletal
- Cancer
- Childhood
- Dental and oral digestive
- Ear, nose and throat
- Endocrine
- Eye and ophthalmologic
- Foot and podiatric
- Genitourinary
- Gynecologic
- Hepatic and biliary
- Immunologic
- Infectious
- Injury and trauma
- Mental
- Metabolic and storage

• Muscular and connective tissue
• Neurologic
• Reproductive
• Respiratory
• Skin and hair

Special sites are provided for:

• Anatomy Explorer
• Calorie Calculator
• Health calculator
• Hospital and Doctor ratings
• Medical encyclopedia
• Medline Search

Netscape: Health
http:www.netscape.com
http://www.health.netscape.com/health/main.tmpl

Health information sites featured include:

• Chats
• Cancer concern
• Diet and nutrition
• Managing stress
• Departments
• Children's health
• Condition centers
• Diet and nutrition
• Emotional health
• Exercise and fitness
• Men's health

- Women's health
- Health Resources
- Ask an expert
- Drug checker
- Medical encyclopedia
- Quit smoking
- What my Dr. reads

Health Search Categories A to Z include:

- Aging
- Alternative medicine
    - Herbs
    - Supplements
    - Vitamins
- Child health
- Conditions and diseases A to Z
- Consumer support groups
- Dentistry
- Disabilities
- Education
- Environmental health
- Fitness
- Healthcare industry
- Health insurance
- Home health
- Medicine
- Men's health
- Nursing
- Nutrition
- Occupational health and safety
- Organizations

- Pharmacy
- Professions
- Public health and safety
- Publications
- Reproductive health
- Resources
- Senior health
- Senses
- Services
- Society/issues/health
- Substance abuse
- Teen's health
- Vision
- Weight loss
- Women's health

NetWellness
http://www.netwellness.org

Netwellness provides quality health information and education services from the University of Cincinnati, Ohio State University and Case Western Reserve University. The subjects include health, wellness, medical, drug, diet, fitness.

- Ask an expert
- Clinical trials
- Health centers
- Health topics
- How to use the information
- Library: offers electronic encyclopedias, patient education materials, handbooks, magazines, and literature databases
- Other health web sites for additional information

- Search for health topics of interest
- Today's news
- What's new

Northern Light
http://www.northernlight.com

Includes search features enabling you to save time while finding out what you want to know about health and wellness. Features custom search, huge web database and advanced search techniques for any health topic of interest.

Pub Med (National Library of Medicine)
http://www.ncbi.nlm.nih.gov/pubmed

PubMed is the National Library of Medicine's search service with access to over 10 million citations on Medline, PreMedline and other related databases, with links to participating online journals. Provides comprehensive consumer information on health and wellness.

Search Engine Databases and Newswires (SEDN)
http://www.internets.com

This web site provides direct access to a large collection of Internet search engines and databases on health and wellness. It has received glowing reviews from the press and universities and subscribes to the Health on the Net Code of Conduct for reliable sites.

MedNets is an international site with proprietary search engines for every specialty in medicine searching only medical databases. Categories include:

- Research engines: search by medical specialty

- Mednets.com: for professionals
- Mednets.org: for patients
- Mednets.net: for health industry

University of Hertfordshire (United Kingdom)
http:hets.ac.uk
http://herts.ac.uk/lis/subjects/health/hlthwww.htm

Contains a list of health information sites relevant to the areas of teaching and research at the University of Hertfordshire, United Kingdom. The list is divided by subject or specialty and has an alphabetical index at the beginning with all information listed and assessed by medical and health professionals.

Ways are presented to the reader to assess the quality of Web health information.

Index of subjects and specialties provided include:

- Aging
- Aids/HIV
- Allergies
- Alternative and complementary therapy
- Alzheimer's disease
- Anatomy and physiology
- Cancer and oncology
- Cardiovascular
- Child health and pediatrics
- Clinical guidelines
- Community care
- Critical care
- Death and euthanasia
- Diabetes and endocrinology
- Diseases and disease classification

- Drug addition and abuse
- Drugs and prescribing
- Elderly
- Electronic journals
- Emergency health services
- Epidemiology
- Family planning
- Gastroenterology
- Geriatrics and aging
- Health and medical computing and software
- Health and medical informatics and information
- Health and medical organizations
- Health economics
- Health management, policy and research
- Health outcomes
- Health promotion
- Health technology assessment
- Imaging
- Infection control
- Learning disabilities
- Medical equipment and devices
- Medical ethics
- Men's health
- Mental health
- Midwifery
- Morbidity and mortality
- Neurosciences
- Nursing
- Nutrition
- Obstetrics and gynecology
- Oncology
- Orthopedics

- Orthotics and prosthetics
- Osteoporosis
- Pediatrics
- Pain management
- Palliative care
- Paramedics
- Pathology
- Pharmacology
- Physiology
- Physiotherapy
- Prescribing
- Primary and community care
- Prosthetics
- Public health
- Radiology and imaging
- Reproductive health
- Respiratory care
- Rheumatology
- Spinal disorders
- Sports medicine
- Statistics
- Telemedicine
- Tissue viability
- Trauma
- Women's health
- World Wide Web health and medical lists
- Wound care

WebCrawler: Health
http://www.webcrawler.com/health

Health information sites featured include:

- Alternative medicine
- Diet and nutrition
- Disabilities
- Diseases and conditions A to Z
- Drugs
- Exercise and fitness
- Family health
- For professionals
- Health headlines from Reuters News/Health Information Services
- Medical encyclopedia
- Medical insurance
- Mental health
- Miscellaneous
- Procedures
- Quick reference
- Search by keyword or browse by topic
- Sexual health
- Support groups
- Talk about health
- Tools and calculators
    - BMI
    - Caloric need
    - Ideal weight
    - More calculators
- Quizzes
    - Asthma I.Q.
    - Cholesterol I.Q
    - Healthy heart I.Q.
    - Heart disease I.Q.

WebMD
http://www.shn.webmd.com

Health, wellness and healthcare sites featured include:

- Health and wellness
  - Dean Ornish, M.D. lifestyle
  - Health-E-tools
  - Living better
  - Sports and fitness
- Home and news
  - Today's live events
  - Health TV
  - My health record
- Living better, smarter, sexier, happier:
- Medical information
  - Clinical trials
  - Diseases and conditions A to Z
  - Drugs and herbs
  - Medical library
  - Self care
- Newly diagnosed: choose a topic
- My healthcare
  - Find a doctor, clinic
  - My health plan
- Quick search for any health topic of interest in all of WebMD, etc.
- WebMD and member services
  - Edit my profile
  - Health risk appraisal
  - Member communities
  - WebMD live events

Wellness Web
http://www.wellweb.com

A leading healthcare resource featuring information in sections on Conventional Medicine, Complementary/Alternative Medicine, and Nutrition and Fitness.

Conventional Medicine section features information on:

- Cancer center
- Cholesterol center
- Diagnostic tests
- Female sex dysfunction
- Fitness center
- Heart center
- Health insurance center
- Impotence center
- Master index of disease and conditions A to Z
- Pain management
- Questionable health practices
- Resources
- Senior center
- Smoker's clinic
- Surgery center
- Wellness centers
- Wellness Web online bookstore
- What's new
- Woman's health center

Complementary and Alternative Medicine section provides information on:

- Cancer prevention
- Herbs and supplements
- Index of diseases, condition and treatments

- Nutritional medicine
- Overview
- Questionable practices
- Resources
- Therapeutic systems and approaches
- What's new
- Women's health

Nutrition and Fitness section includes information on:

- Carbohydrates, protein and fat
- Eating disorders
- Eating out
- Food safety
- Healthy meals and snacks
- Herbs, vitamins and mineral supplements
- Nutrition and aging
- Nutrition and diet
- Nutrition and disease
- Nutrition and pregnancy
- Nutrition for children and adolescents
- Overview of nutrition
- Questionable diet and nutrition practices
- Recommendations
- Required nutrients
- Resources
- Sports and nutrition
- What's fun/what's interesting
- What's new in nutrition
- Vegetarianism
- Weight management

Yahoo: Health
http://www.yahoo.com/health
http://dir.yahoo.com/health/diseases_and_conditions
http://dir.yahoo.com/health/web_directories
http://dir.yahoo.com/health/mental_health/counseling_and_ther-apy/ therapeutic_methods

Yahoo provides health research, expert advice, healthy recipes and more. Categories of health information provided include:

• Alternative medicine
• Chats and forums
• Children's health
• Conferences
• Death and dying
• Dentistry
• Disabilities
• Diseases and conditions
• Education
• Emergency services
• Environmental health
• First aid
• Fitness
• General health
• Health administration
• Health care
• Health sciences
• Hospitals and medical centers
• Institutes
• Law
• Long term care
• Medicine

- Men's health
- Mental health
- Midwifery
- News and media
- Nursing
- Nutrition
- Organizations
- Pharmacy
- Procedures and therapies
- Public health and safety
- Reference
- Reproductive health
- Senior health
- Sexuality
- Teen's health
- Traditional medicine
- Travel health and medicine
- Web directories
- Weight issues
- Women's health
- Workplace

Diseases and conditions information featured includes:

- Allergies
- Anxiety disorders
- Autoimmune disease
- Back and neck injuries
- Birth defects
- Blood disorders bone disease
- Brain and spinal diseases
- Cancer

• Circulation diseases
• Dental conditions
• Depressive disorders
• Digestion and nutrition disorders
• Dissociative disorder
• Ear conditions
• Eating disorders
• Eye conditions
• Food allergies
• Foodborne illnesses
• Genetic disorders
• Heart diseases
• Hormonal disorders
• Impulse control disorders
• Infectious diseases
• Institutes
• Intestinal diseases
• Kidney disease
• Language disorders
• Leukodystrophies
• Liver disease
• Mental health
• Metabolic diseases
• Mood disorders
• Neurological diseases
• Organizations
• Personality disorders
• Pregnancy complications
• Prion disease
• Registries
• Respiratory diseases
• Skin conditions

- Sleep disorders
- Sports injuries
- Tropical diseases
- Vestibular disorders

Chapter V

Health Categories, Diseases, Resources, and Web Sites

Information in this section is organized into an alphabetical list of over 100 categories of health information. Each category contains an alphabetical list of key Web sites. Information from one or more of the following types of Search Tools listed below is provided for each health category.
- Commercial Search Engines
- Medical Colleges/Schools/Universities
- Professional Medical Societies
- Professional Organizations
- US Government Sources

Not all Search Tool Resources that may have information pertaining to the category of health information of interest are provided under the various health categories and diseases covered in this Chapter. Therefore, in searching for healthcare information pertaining to any given health category, topic, or disease, you need to review whatever information may be offered via the various Search Tools listed in Chapter IV and use those most appropriate for desired information before reaching any definitive conclusions regarding information available on the Web.

Eugene A. DeFelice, M.D. • 115

Health Categories, Diseases, Resources and Web Sites

Aging and Geriatrics
Acupuncture and Oriental Medicine
Alcoholism
Allergy
Alternative, Complimentary, Natural, and Herbal Medicine
Alzheimer's Disease
American Medical Association
Arthritis
Association of American Medical Colleges
Autoimmune and Immune Disorders
Blood Disorders
British Medical Journal
Cancer
Cardiovascular Disease (Heart and Blood Vessels)
Chest and Lung Disorders
Child Health and Safety (Pediatrics)
Clinical Trials
Colorblindness
Colds and Flu
Dartmouth Atlas of Health Care
Death and Dying, Hospice and Palliative Medicine
Dental and Craniofacial Disorders
Diabetes Mellitus
Dietary Guidelines: Revision 2000
Dietary Supplements and Vitamins
Digestive Disorders (Gastrointestinal)
Disabilities
Disease Control and Prevention
Doctor's Guide to the Internet

Drugs and Medications
Ear, Nose and Throat Disorders (Otolaryngology)
Eating Disorders
Endocrine Disorders
Environmental Health and Safety
Epilepsy
Eye Disorders
Family Medicine and Health
Fitness, Diet, and Exercise
Genetic Disorders
Harvard Medical Center
Headache
Healthcare Research and Quality
Health Insurance
Hearing
Home Health
Hospitals
Human Anatomy
Hypertension
Hypnosis
Industrial and Occupational Health
Infectious Disease
Internal Medicine
Journal of the American Medical Association
Kidney Disease
Lancet
Leukemias and Lymphomas
Medical Colleges/Schools
Medical Dictionary and Medical Encyclopedia
Meditation
Medline
Medlineplus

Men's Health
Mental Health
Mental Retardation
Merck Manual
Musculoskeletal and Orthopedic Disorders
National Institutes of Health Institutes and Centers
National Library of Medicine
Neurological Disorders
New England Journal of Medicine
Nuclear Medicine
Nutrition, Food and Health
Obesity and Weight Control
Occupational Health and Safety
Orthopedic Disorders
Otolaryngology Disorders (Ear, Nose Throat)
Pain
Parkinson's Disease
Pediatric Disorders
Physical Medicine and Rehabilitation
Physicians and Professional Organizations
Planned Parenthood
Podiatry and Foot Disorders
Practice Guidelines
Preventive Medicine
Psychology and Counseling
Public Health and Consumer Medicine
Radiology
Rare Disorders
Reproductive Medicine
Sexually Transmitted Disease
Skin Disorders (Dermatology)
Sleep Disorders

Sports Medicine and Sports Disorders
Statistical Health Resources
Stress
Stroke
Suicide and Prevention
Surgery
Transplantation
Travel Health
Urological Disorders
Vaccines and Immunization Schedules
Veteran's Health
Violence Prevention
Vitamins
Wellness
Women's Health

Health Categories, Diseases, Resources and Web Sites

Aging and Geriatrics

➤ American Geriatrics Society
http://www.americangeriatrics.org

Information on aging, news, education, public policy, AGS Foundation for Health in Aging, and health inks to other resources.

➤ Baylor College of Medicine (Huffington Center on Aging)
http://www.bcm.tmc.edu/hcoa

Focuses on research, healthcare for older people and education of health professionals and consumers.
➤ Gerontological Society of America

http://www.geron.org

Aging information, news, interest groups, publications, online resources, and search for any aging topic of interest

➢ National Institute of Aging
   http://www.nih.gov/nia

Leading Federal effort on aging, health information, research programs, prevention, news and events. Search aging topics of interest via NIA search site.

➢ National Senior Citizens Law Center
   http://www.nsclc.org

Advocates, litigates, and publishes on low income elderly and disability issues including Medicare, Medicaid, Social Security, nursing homes, age discrimination and pensions.

Acupuncture and Oriental Medicine

➢ National Acupuncture and Oriental Medicine Alliance
   http://www.acuall.org

An alliance of practitioners and consumers working to advance acupuncture and oriental medicine. Features information on:
   • Acupuncture Alliance
   • Acupuncture and oriental medicine treatment
   • Conferences and workshops
   • General information on acupuncture and oriental medicine
   • Legislative status
   • National professional issues

> • Publications of interest
> • Qualified practitioners in your area

➤ National Center for Complementary and Alternative Medicine
  http://www.nccam.nih.gov

NCCAM is the leading Federal center regarding information on acupuncture and oriental medicine. Provides health information, research programs, treatment, and news and events. Search acupuncture and oriental medicine topics of interest.

Alcoholism

➤ Alcoholic Anonymous
  http://www.alcoholics-anonymous.org

  Serves the U.S. and Canada. Information provided on:

  • About AA
  • AA fact file
  • AA grapevine
  • Anonymity letter to media
  • Do you think you are different
  • Information for professionals
  • Intergroups and answering services
  • International convention
• International general offices
• Is AA for you
• Is there an alcoholic in your life
• Message to teenagers
• Newcomer asks
• Questions and answers

• US/Canada Central Offices

➤ National Council on Alcoholism and Drug Dependence (NCAAD)
  http://www.ncadd.net

Advocates prevention, intervention, research, and treatment of alcoholism and other drug addictions. Features information on:

> • Advocacy
> • Affiliates
> • Awareness activities
> • Campaign to prevent kids from drinking
> • Definition of alcoholism
> • Facts about alcoholism and other drug addictions
> • Health information
> • History of NCADD

• National intervention network
• News
• Online communications center
• Parents information
• Prevention and treatment programs
• Publications
• Registry of addiction recovery
• Resource and referral guide
• Youth information

➤ National Institute on Alcohol Abuse and Alcoholism
  http://www.niaaa.nih.gov

Leading U.S. Government effort regarding alcoholism, health information, research programs, treatment, prevention and news and events. Search any alcoholism topic of interest via the NIAAA search engine.

➤ Rational Recovery Systems
    http://www.rational.org/recovery

Self-help system of planned abstinence via a learned thinking skill called Addictive Voice Recognition Technique (AVRT).

Allergy

➤ American Academy of Allergy, Asthma and Immunology
    http://www.aaaai.org

Provides information on allergy, allergic diseases, diagnosis, prevention and treatment. Features sites on:

- All about allergies, pollen and spore counts
- Allergy and asthma
- Exercise-induced asthma
- Immunotherapy
- Media and news information
- Meetings
- Patient and public resources
- Pediatric asthma
- Physician referral directory
- Publications
- Seniors and asthma
- Sinusitis
- Tips to remember

➤ American College of Allergy, Asthma and Immunology
    http://www.allergy.mcg.edu

Maintained by allergists and medical specialists who treat allergies and asthma. Provides information on allergy including medical news and an allergist locator.

➢ Asthma and Allergy Foundation of America
  http://www.aafa.org

  Features sites on:
    • Action against asthma
    • Asthma and allergy information
    • Asthma and allergy news
    • Ask the allergist
    • Check your local pollen count
    • Free asthma screenings
  • Health professionals
  • Kids and teens
  • Medical assistance programs
  • Search on asthma or allergy topics of interest

➢ National Institute of Allergy and Infectious Disease
  http://www.niaid.nih.gov

Leading Federal effort regarding allergy and infectious disease. Provides information on allergy prevention, treatment, research, news and events. Search on allergy topics of interest via the NIAID search engine.

Alternative, Complementary, Natural and Herbal Medicine

➢ Alternative Medicine Homepage (AMH)
  http://www.pitt.edu/~cbw/altm.html

AMH is sponsored by the University of Pittsburgh and provides information on "unconventional, unorthodox, unproven, alternative, complementary, innovative and integrative therapies... Since 1996, the National Library of Medicine and the MeSH(medical subject headings) Term Working Group, Office of Alternative Medicine, National Institutes of Health classifies alternative medicine as an unrelated group of nonorthodox therapeutic practices, often with explanatory systems that do not follow conventional medical or biomedical explanations. The National Library of Medicine's previous classification was non-orthodox therapeutic systems that have no satisfactory scientific explanation for their reported effectiveness. Alternative therapies include but are not limited to herbal medicine, diet fads, homeopathy, faith and spiritual healing, new age healing, chiropractic, acupuncture, naturopathy, massage, aromatherapy, and music therapy. AMH provides links to Internet information sources and does not replace treatment by a qualified health practitioner." Sites featured include:

- AIDS/HIV
- Databases
- Directories
- Government/Pennsylvania related resources
- Internet resources
- Practitioners

➤ American Botanical Council
   http://www.herbalgram.org
   http://www.herbalgram.org/commission_e/index.html

"Dedicated to the safe and effective use of medicinal plants/herbs and educating the public and government agencies, research institutions and industry on sold scientific research that can guide decisions about producing and consuming herbal/plant based products that may benefit health. Monograms produced by ABC are reported to represent among the most accurate information available on the safety and efficacy of herbs and phytomedicines, including a glossary of anatomical, botanical, medical, pharmaceutical and technical terms. The Complete German Commission E Monographs entitled "Therapeutic Guide to Herbal Medicines" as well as the more recent "Herbal Medicine" are available in English."

➤ National Center for Complementary Alternative Medicine
  http://www.nccam.nih.gov

Chief U.S. Government effort regarding complementary alternative medicine information, research, treatment, news and events. Search any alternative, complementary, natural, herbal medicine topic of interest via the NCCAM search site.

➤ Natural Medicines Comprehensive Database
  http://www.naturaldatabase.com

Extensive information on herbal medicines and dietary supplements used in the Western World. Compiled by pharmacists and physicians who are part of the Pharmacist's Letter and Prescriber Letter research editorial staff. They evaluate natural medicines by the same medical criteria that are used to evaluate prescription and non-prescription drugs. Believed to be one of the most extensive, scientific and practical databases on natural medicines available anywhere. Search features are provided to find use, efficacy, adverse effects, interactions and safety of each natural medicine. Must subscribe and pay a fee for use.

Alzheimer's Disease

➤ Alzheimer's.com
  http://www.alzheimers.com

Provides practical, current information to empower Alzheimer's caregivers to manage the disease more effectively.

➤ Alzheimer's Disease Education and Referral Center
http://www.alzheimers.org/adear

Latest news from the National Institute on Aging about Alzheimer's Disease, research, symptoms, diagnosis, treatment, drug trials, services for patient and families and professional meetings

➤ Alzheimer's Research Foundation
http://www.alzheimer's_research.org

Privately funded organization offering current information, news and Internet sources regarding the disorder.

➤ National Institute of Aging (NIA)
http://www.nih.gov/nia

Chief Federal effort concerning health and aging and Alzheimer's Disease. Provides information on diagnosis, research, treatment, news and events. Use NIA search site for Alzheimer's Disease information of interest.

American Medical Association
http://www.ama-assn.org
http://www.ama-assn.org/about/guidelines.htm
http://www.ama-assn.org/consumer/gnrl.htm
http://www.ama-assn.org/special/womh.htm

Reliable information provided on vast majority of health topics. Use AMA search site for health information and resources. AMA guidelines are provided for searching the Web for health information.

Arthritis

➤ American College of Rheumatology (ACR)
   http://www.rheumatology.org/index.asp

Provides arthritis research publications and other information. Use ACR's search site to obtain information on arthritis topics of interest. Enhanced search capabilities include keyword, author and title search of available issues of their official journal, *Arthritis and Rheumatism*, online. Cross-journal searching between the journal, *Arthritis Care and Research* also is available.

➤ Arthritis Foundation
   http://www.arthritis.org

   Features sites for:

      • Advocacy groups
      • Arthritis feature of the day
      • Arthritis questions and answers
   • Arthritis topic search
   • Read Arthritis Today

➤ American Juvenile Arthritis Organization
   http://www.arthritis.org/answers/about_ajao.asp

   Relevant information on juvenile arthritis.

➤ Medlineplus
   http://www.nlm.nih.gov/medlineplus/arthritis.htm

Provides access to arthritis information available through the National Library of Medicine primarily for consumers and patients.

Association of American Medical Colleges (AAMC)
http://www.aamc.org

Health site features following information:
- AAMC Member Academic and Professional Societies: alphabetical listing and listing by discipline
- AAMC Member Teaching Hospitals and Health Systems: alphabetical listing, geographical listing and Medicare provider numbers
- Medical Education site provides AAMC list of medical schools

Academic and professional societies, teaching hospitals and health systems, and medical schools listed provide a wide range of health information. To obtain Web sites, type the name of the academic or professional society or medical school in the search site provided on any search engine and you will be directed to the appropriate Web site address.

Autoimmune and Immune Disorders

➢ American Academy of Allergy, Asthma, and Immunology
　http://www.aaaai.org

➢ American Association of Immunologists
　http://www.aai/default.asp
➢ American College of Allergy, Asthma and Immunology
　http://www.allergy.mcg.edu

Above 3 resources provide relevant information on autoimmune and immune disorders.

➢ American Autoimmune Related Disease Association
  http://www.aarda.org

Patient information on over 56 autoimmune-related diseases. Features articles from their newsletter *Women and Autoimmunity*, research reports, helpful tips for coping with autoimmune disease as well as links to other resources.

➢ National Institute of Allergy and Infectious Diseases
  http://www.niaid.nih.gov

Features information sites on:

  • Acquired immunodeficiency
  • Allergy
  • Immunology
• Search for information on autoimmune and immune disorders topics of interest
• Transplantation

Blood Disorders

➢ American Society of Hematology
  http://www.hematology.org

Information on blood disorders by clinicians and scientists committed to advancing the understanding, prevention, diagnosis and treatment of hematologic disorders including diseases of the blood, bone marrow, immunologic, and hemostatic systems. Features official journal, *Blood*, educational materials, international outreach resources and patient group links.

➤ American Society Pediatric Hematology and Oncology
  http://www.aspho.org

Pediatric hematologists who study and treat childhood cancer and
blood diseases. Features sites for official journal, online resources and
what's new.

➤ Leukemia and Lymphoma Society
  http://www.leukemia_lymphoma.org

Provides information and supports research regarding blood related
cancers such as leukemia, lymphoma, multiple myeloma and other disorders. Supports patients and their families as they cope with the daily chal-
lenges of blood related cancers by providing relevant information and
guidance and support nationally as well as through a local network of 57
chapters. Currently supports over 360 researchers doing basic and trans-
lational research into better understanding, treatment and cures for
leukemia, lymphoma and myeloma. Sites are provided for:

> • Local chapter finder
> • Patients and family
> • Public and press
- • Researchers and professionals
- • What's new in research

➤ National Heart, Lung and Blood Institute (NHLBI)
  http://www.nhbli.nih.gov/health/public/blood/index.html

Premier Federal effort concerning blood disorders. Features information sites on:

> • Blood transfusion and safety

- Hemophilia
  - Raynaud's phenomena
- Thrombocytopenia purpura
- What's new in blood disorders

Publications on blood disorders are available. Refer to National Cancer Institute for additional information on cancers of the blood. Use NHLBI search site to obtain other information on blood disorders of interest.

British Medical Journal

➤ British Medical Journal (BMJ)
  http://www.bmj.com
  http://www.bmj.com/collections

One of the premier medical journals published in the United Kingdom. Collections of BMJ articles are made available by specialty and topic. From an extensive list, click on specialty or topic to obtain details of all relevant articles on the subjects published by BMJ since January 1998. Topics featured include:

- Anesthesia
- Cardiovascular medicine
- Complementary medicine
- Critical care and intensive care
- Dentistry and oral medicine
- Dermatology
- Drugs
- Emergency medicine
- Endocrinology
- Evidence based practice
- Gastroenterology

- General practice, family practice and primary care
- Genetics
- Geriatric medicine
- Obstetrics and gynecology
- Renal medicine
- Immunology
- Infectious disease
- Medicine in developing countries
- Molecular medicine
- Neurology
- Newsworthy disease and disorders
- Nutrition and metabolism
- Occupational health
- Oncology (cancer)
- Palliative medicine
- Pathology
- Pediatrics
- Physiotherapy
- Prison medicine
- Psychiatry
- Rehabilitation medicine
- Respiratory medicine
- Rheumatology
- Sexual medicine
- Sports medicine
- Surgery
- Travel medicine

Cancer

➢ American Cancer Society
  http://www.cancer.org

Dedicated to helping those who face cancer, through research, early detection, education, treatment and other patient services.

➤ American Society of Pediatric Hematology and Oncology
   http://www.aspo.org

Information and research related to pediatric hematology and oncology and cancer prevention and control.

➤ Breast Cancer Research
   http://www.breast-cancer-research.com

Array of breast disease and cancer information sites and links.

➤ Cancer Care
   http://www.cancercareinc.org

Online support groups, referrals, and toll free counseling line. Free professional help to people with all types of cancer through counseling, education, information, referrals and direct financial assistance, if necessary. Special sections are provided on a variety of common cancers. You may obtain cancer information of interest via their search site.

➤ Leukemia and Lymphoma Society
   http://www.leukemia_lymphoma.org

Resource for patients with leukemia or lymphoma.

➤ National Cancer Institute (NCI)
   http://www.nci.nih.gov

Leading U.S. Government effort regarding cancer, risk factors, types, diagnosis, treatment, publications and reports, news and statistics. Further information on cancer topics of interest is available via NCI search site.

➢ Oncolink (University of Pennsylvania School of Medicine Cancer Center)
  http://www.oncolink.upenn.edu

Premier cancer information web site. Provides information on a wide variety of cancers, their causes, prevention and treatment. Sites featured include:
> • Abramson Family Cancer Research Institute
> • Book reviews
> • Cancer causes, screening and prevention
> • Cancer news
> • Clinical trials
> • Conferences and meetings
> • Different medical and surgical specialties involved
* Editor's choice topics
* Frequently asked questions and answers
* Global resource for cancer information
* Oncolink
* Psychosocial support and personal experiences
* Specific types of cancer
* Symptom management

Further information on cancer topics of interest is available via search site provided.

Cardiovascular Disease (Heart and Blood Vessels)

➤ American College of Cardiology (ACC)
http://www.acc.org

Heart disease is the leading cause of death, for both men and women,
killing around three quarters of a million Americans each year. As many as
two thirds of the heart disease deaths may be preventable. ACC is a lead-
ing professional organization involved in the prevention and treatment of
heart disease. Information sites featured include:
- Clinical information/guidelines
- Frequently asked questions and answers
- *Journal American College Cardiology* online
- News on cardiology
- Patient education
- Search for information on cardiology topics of interest

➤ American Heart Association (AHA)
http://www.americanheart.org

Extensive information on heart and other cardiovascular disorders provided for professionals and public via following sites:

- American Stroke Association for stroke prevention, treatment
and recovery
- Family health, nutrition and exercise
- Heart and stroke A to Z guide
- Meetings and councils
- Research
- Science and professional publications
- Statistics
- Warning signs
- What's your risk
- Your heart, disease, condition and treatment

Further topic searches include *Search the AHA Web*, which includes several ways to find what you are looking for; *Search for*, which is the AHA search site for specific topics and information of interest; and finally you can go to Heart and Stroke A to Z Guide to find direct links to commonly requested information.

➤ International Society for Heart and Lung Transplantation
http://www.ishlt.org

Features general information, annual transplant registry, board and committee results, heart failure registry, programs and services and transplant notification entry.

➤ Istituto Mario Negri (Milan, Italy)
http://www.irfmn.mnegri.it

Premier Italian institute which provides extensive cardiovascular disease and other health information. Click on Cardio.care for information on cardiac failure, cardiovascular disease prevention, hypertension, myocardial infarction, peripheral arteriography, stroke, venous thromboembolic disease and ventricular arrhythmias, etc. Access to a variety of electronic journals, cardiovascular databases and other links are provided.

➤ National Heart, Lung and Blood Institute
http://www.nhlbi.nih.gov
http://www.nhlbi.nih.gov/health/prof/heart/index.htm
http://www.nhlbi.nih.gov/health/public/heart/index.htm

Leading U.S. government effort regarding information on cardiovascular disorders, research, diagnosis and treatment, clinical trials, publications and news. You may use their search site to obtain information on cardiovascular disorder topics of interest.

Chest and Lung Disorders

➤ American College of Chest Physicians
  http://www.chestnet.org

Clinical information on chest disorders, news and links. Online publications include:

- Chest Soundings
- Chest 2000
- Experience-based practice guidelines
- Patient education guides
- Pulmonary Perspectives
- Search for information on chest disorder topics of interest

➤ American Lung Association
  http://www.lungusa.org

ALA features information on:

- Advocacy efforts
- Air quality
- Ask ALA
- Asthma
- Data and statistics
- Diseases and condition A to Z
- Learn about your lungs
- Livings with lung disease
- Local ALA programs and events
- Occupational health
- Research
- Search for lung topics of interest

      • School programs
      • Tobacco control

➤ National Heart, Lung and Blood Institute
   http://www.nhlbi.nih.gov/health/public/lung/index.htm
   http://www.nhlbi.nih.gov/health/prof/lung/index.htm

Leading Federal effort regarding lung disease, diagnosis, treatment, research, clinical trials, publications and what's new/news. Use search site provided to obtain information on chest/lung disease topics of interest.

➤ University of Maryland School of Medicine (Thoracic Surgery Division)
   http://www. umm.edu/thoracic

The Thoracic Surgery Division is nationally recognized center for developing innovative treatments for disorders of the structures and organs of the chest, particularly the lungs. Played a leading role in the development and use of visually-assisted thoracoscopic surgery which is reported to be less invasive and involving fewer complications. Offers this minimally invasive technique to treat hyperhydrosis (excessive sweating) via thoracoscopic sympathectomy. Also, emphysema may be treated via a rehabilitation program and/or lung volume reduction therapy.

Child Health and Safety (Pediatrics)

➤ American Academy for Cerebral Palsy and Developmental Medicine
   http://www.aacpdm.org

Health professionals, parents and patients can begin their online research in these fields and topics of interest, by clicking on to the Library Section.

➤ American Academy of Pediatrics
  http://www.aap.org

Fosters the attainment of optimal physical, mental and social health and well being for all infants, children, adolescents and young adults. Provides information on advocacy, research, you and your family, education, publications and news on pediatrics. Search any pediatric disorder of interest via the site provided.

➤ American Cleft Palate and Craniofacial Association
  http://www.cleft.org

Information on cleft palate and craniofacial disorders.

➤ Dr. Greene.com
  http://www.drgreene.com

Pediatric information following via sites:

- Ask a question
- Allergies
- Bedwetting
- Breast feeding
- Diseases and Conditions A to Z
- Ear infections
- Eating and nutrition
- Genetics
- HIV and AIDS

- Immunizations
- Infectious disease
- Parenting
- Potty training
- Rashes
- Safety
- Search for pediatric health topics
- Sleep

➤ Kid's Health
   http://www.kidshealth.org

Created by Nemours Foundation, Kids Health.org provides an array of information on children's health, infections, behavior and emotions, food and fitness and growing up healthy.

➤ National Academy for Child Development
   http://www.nacd.org

International organization of parents and professionals dedicated to helping infants, children and young adults to reach their full potential. Designs home neuro-developmental programs for clients with disorders and conditions such as:

- Attention Deficit Disorder
- Autism
- Brain injured
- Cerebral palsy
- Comatose
- Developmentally delayed
- Distractible
- Down syndrome

- Dyslexic
- Fetal alcohol syndrome
- Fragile X
- Gifted
- Hyperactive
- Learning disabled
- Minimal brain dysfunction
- PDD
- Retarded
- Rett Syndrome
- Tourette's Syndrome
- William's Syndrome

Provides information sites for:

- Feature and other articles
- Journal
- Products
- Programs
- Research
- Resources
- Search for child development topics of interest
- What's new

➤ National Down Syndrome Society
  http://www.ndss.org

Online information source about Down Syndrome via sites provided on:

- About Down Syndrome
- Advocacy
- Affiliates

•Events and conferences
•Information and referral services
- Publications
- Questions and answers
- Web links
- What's new

➤ National Institute of Child Health and Human Development
http://www.nichd.nih.gov

Premier U.S. Government effort regarding child health and human development, research, treatment, clinical trials, news and publications. Use search site provided to obtain information on child health, safety and development topics of interest.

➤ Society for Adolescent Medicine
http://www.adolescenthealth.org

Information on adolescent health and wellness.

➤ United Cerebral Palsy Association
http://www.ucpa.org

Useful information for health professionals, parents and patients regarding cerebral palsy.

Clinical Trials

➤ Center Watch Clinical Trials Listing Service
http://www.centerwatch.com

National and international listing of clinical trials in all therapeutic areas. Resources include:

- Additional resources for industry professionals and patients
- Background information on clinical research
- Clinical trial notification service
- CW publications
- Industry news
- Listing of clinical trials
- Newly FDA approved therapies
- NIH studies
- Patient advocates
- Research center profiles
- Research headlines

➢ Search Clinical Research Studies Database
   http://www.clinicalstudies.info.nih.gov

Collection of research clinical trials being conducted at the National Institutes of Health Clinical Center. Enter the diagnosis, sign or symptom or other key word or phrases. Full-text search including and excluding eligibility criteria and browse by institute of the principal investigator and primary disease category. Frequently asked questions and answers site is available.

➢ National Institutes of Health Clinical Center
   http://www.cc.nih.gov

Clinical trials open to select patients at the National Institute of Health Clinical Center.

Colorblindness

➤ Ask a Biologist
   http://www.askabiologist.asu.edu/research/seecolor/colortest.html

Color blindness test created by Arizona State University's Life Sciences Visualization Group and designed for students and teachers of Grades K through 12. A set of 5 Ishihara test charts is provided along with brief, straightforward explanations about color blindness. Information is presented clearly and succinctly and terms defined throughout the site. Links are provided for more information on colorblindness.

➤ Google Web Directory: Health
   http://www.directory.google.com/top/health

Click on color blindness-information and tests of interest. You will find Ask a Biologist color blindness test in the list of tests provided.

➤ National Eye Institute
   http://www.nei.nih.gov

Use search site to obtain information on colorblindness.

Colds and Flu
http://www.4colds4anything.com
http://www.4flu4anything.com
Two useful web sites dealing with the common cold and the flu. 4cold4anything.com offers general information about the common cold, how one catches it, and a critical view about over-the-counter cold medicines. 4flu4anything.com provides flu information orientation and treatment and alternative medicines plus a look at "home remedies" from "the Chinese Medicine Cabinet". Vaccines and prescription medicine information are provided.

Dartmouth Atlas of Health Care
http://www.dartmouthatlas.org

Healthcare decision making information for patients and their physicians. Published by the Center for Evaluative Clinical Sciences at Dartmouth Medical School. Since 1966, eighteen (18) editions of the Dartmouth Atlas have been published, including three national editions and nine regional atlases. In 1999, new atlases were published on the treatment of cardiovascular, musculoskeletal and peripheral vascular disease. Among others, reports of interest include:
- 1998 Chapter 5: The Surgical Treatment of Common Disease
- 1999 Chapter 5: Practice Variations and Quality of Surgical Care for Common Conditions?
- 1999 Chapter 7: The Quality of Medical Care in the United States

The 1999 Chapter 7: Quality of Medical Care in the United States and the 1999 Chapter 5: the Surgical Treatment of Common Disease are good places for the patient to begin to become informed. Also, sites featured for further information include:

- About the Atlas
- Major Findings
- Related Research
- Topic Index
- Atlases and Reports
- Archives
- Current Atlases
- Online Reports
- Data Access
- Custom Reports
- Download
- Web Site

• Search for further information of interest

Death and Dying, Hospice and Palliative Medicine

➢ American Academy of Hospice and Palliative Medicine (AAHPM)
  http://www.aahpm.org

The AAHPM is dedicated to the advancement of hospice and palliative medicine, its practice, research and education. This site provides information on AAHPM, events and meetings, links, members' services, products and publications and a search site for obtaining additional material on hospice and palliative medicine topics of interest.

➢ Death and Dying.com
  http://www.death_dying.com/terminalillness
  http://death_dying.com/gentle/planner.html

Information on a wide range of key topics including:

> • Alternative medicine/health
> • Care guide
> • Dying Person's Guide to Dying
> • Legal issues
> • Loss of a loved one

• Medical information
• Pain information
• Planners
• Terminal illness planner

➢ Hospice Net
  http://www.hospicenet.org

Features information sites on:

- Bereavement
- Caregivers
- Dying Person's Guide
- Hospice
- Patients
- Palliative care

➤ Librarians' Index to the Internet
http://www.lii.org

Click on Health and go to site on Death and Dying for available information.

➤ MedExplorer
http://www.medexplorer.com

Go to site provided on Death and Dying.

Dental and Craniofacial Disorders

➤ American Academy of Peridontology
http://www.perio.org

Current information on peridontal disorders.

- Find a periodontologist
- Frequently asked questions and answers
- Journal of Peridontology
- Mouth and body connection
- Periodontal procedures

- Protecting your oral health
- Search for information on topics of interest
- Web links
- What are periodontal diseases
- Your oral health

➤ American Dental Association (ADA)
   http://www.ada.org
   http://www.ada.org/tc-clin.html

ADA provides useful information on a variety of dental topics including:

- ADA Health Foundation
- ADA Library Services
- Dental products and procedures
- Fluorides and fluoridation
- Infection control
- *Journal of the American Dental Association*
- Periodontal disease
- Research issues of importance to the practicing dentist
- Tobacco and nicotine

➤ Harvard School of Dental Medicine
   http://www.hsdm.med.harvard.edu

Harvard School of Dental Medicine is a leading provider of useful dental information. Go to Harvard Dental Center, click on Consumer Dental Education and then click on Common Dental Procedures for information on over 50 topics of common interest. Since the Harvard School of Dental Medicine considers the Internet to be an excellent source for dental information, they share some Web links that they feel are particularly good.

➢ National Institute of Dental and Craniofacial Research
  http://www.nih.gov/cranio/disease/ac.html
  http://www.nih.gov/news/publica.htm
  http://www.nih.gov/news/index.html

Leading U.S. Government provider of dental and craniofacial disorders information. Use Search site to obtain information of interest.

Diabetes Mellitus

➢ American Diabetes Association
  http://www.diabetes.org

Resource for diabetes information with everything you need to know from nutrition to exercise, who's at risk for diabetes, and treatment. Provides the latest news stories on diabetes and consumer magazines and professional journals on the subject. Highlights clinical practice guidelines, recommendations and research for professionals. Advocacy information, legal issues and Internet resources also are available.

➢ Diabetes.com
  http://www.diabetes.com

Online community for diabetics. Includes information sites on diet and exercise, intimacy, risk factors, prevention, and information on symptoms.

➢ Diabetes Control Center
  http://www.dr-diabetes.com

Tips on diabetes and its control by Charles H. Raine, M.D.

➢ Doctor's Guide to the Internet (Diabetes)

http://www.pslgroup.com
http://www.pslgroup.com/diabetes

Guide to diabetes related information and resources likely to be of interest to medical professionals and/or patients.

➤ Endocrine Society
http://www.endo-society.org

Information on Types I and II (adult onset) diabetes.

➤ National Institute Diabetes and Digestive and Kidney Diseases
http://www.niddk.nih.gov

Premier U.S. Government site for information on diabetes mellitus. Features sites on diabetes, nutrition, weight loss and diabetes control and National Diabetes Educational Program. Use search site to obtain further information on diabetes mellitus topics of interest.

Dietary Guidelines: Revision 2000
http://www.americanheart.org
http://www.americanheart.org/dietaryguidelines/index.html

New American Heart Association Dietary Guidelines Revision 2000, designed to help most Americans prevent heart diseases, hypertension and stroke. A statement from healthcare professionals from the Nutrition Committee of the American Heart Association. A more individualized approach to dietary guidelines for patients is provided.

Dietary Supplements and Vitamins

➤ American Medical Association (AMA)

http://www.ama-assn.org
http://www,ana-assn.org/consumer/gnrl.htm

Current information on dietary supplements/vitamins. Go to Consumer Health and click on Supplements, Herbs or Vitamins for available information. Use AMA search site to obtain further information.

➤ Food and Drug Administration (FDA)
http://www.fda.gov
http://www.fda.gov/medwatch

FDA provides current, reliable information on the efficacy, safety and side effects of dietary supplements that may or may not be approved for clinical use. Medwatch provides information about other people's good and bad experiences with supplements (as well as particular brands). You can log in and report adverse effects from dietary supplements via this site.

➤ National Center for Complementary and Alternative Medicine
http://www.nccam.nih.gov

Current, reliable, comprehensive information on dietary supplements including potentially toxic or deadly herbs.

➤ Natural Medicines Comprehensive Database
http://www.naturaldatabase.com

Comprehensive database which includes information about supplement safety, effectiveness, adverse reactions with other drugs and supplements. This site requires a yearly subscription fee for full information.

Digestive Disorders (Gastrointestional)

➢ American College of Gastroenterology
  http://www.acg.gi.org

  Features information on:

  • *American Journal of Gastroenterology*
  • Clinical updates
  • Colon cancer
  • Common Gastrointestinal problems
  • Digestive health tips
  • Gastrointestinal physician locator
  • Other resources
  • Patient education brochures

➢ American Gastroenterological Association
  http://www.gastro.org

  Public section and search sites provide information on a wide variety of gastrointestinal disorders as well as:

  • Educational articles
  • Publications
  • What's new

➢ American Liver Foundation
  http://www.liverfoundation.org

  Information on liver disorders and advocacy groups.

➢ American Society for Gastrointestional Endoscopy
  http://www.asge.org

Gastroenterologists, surgeons, and other digestive health specialists committed to furthering the knowledge, diagnosis, and treatment of digestive disorders through the appropriate use of endoscopic techniques. You may view the online database of clinical updates, patient care guidelines, policy and position statements and search the database of members to find an endoscopist in your area.

➤ Crohn's and Colitis Foundation of America
   http://www.ccfa.org

Current information on Crohn's disease and colitis.

➤ Digestive Health Resource Center
   http://www.gastro.org/public/digestinfo.html

Information and resources on digestive disorders.

➤ Hepatitis Foundation International
   http://www.hepfi.org

Features information sites on:

   • Alerts about hepatitis
   • Caring for your liver
   • Diagnosis of hepatitis
   • Treatment of hepatitis
   • Vaccination against hepatitis

➤ International Foundation for Functional Gastroentestinal Disorders
   http://www.iffgd.org

Focuses on Irritable Bowel Syndrome. Features sites for information on:

- Functional disorders of the esophagus (gastroesophageal reflux disease or GERD), heartburn, non cardiac chest pain, Barrett's esophagus)
- Bowel disorders (irritable bowel syndrome, constipation, diarrhea, bloating, gas, abdominal pain)
- Gastroduodenal disorders (dyspepsia, nausea, upper abdominal pain)
- Intestinal malabsorption syndrome
- Rectal and anal disorders (anal and rectal discomfort, dysfunction and pain, anal fistulas, proctitis, anal fissure)
- Pelvic muscle dysfunction (incontinence, etc)
- Pelvic pain

➤ National Institute of Diabetes and Digestive and Kidney Diseases
http://www.niddk.nih.gov

Premier Federal effort and resource on a wide variety of digestive and nutritional disorders. Use the search site provided for information on digestive disorders of interest.

Disabilities

➤ American Academy of Disability Evaluating Physicians
http://www.aadep.org/intro.htm

Information regarding disability evaluating physicians.

➤ Google Web Directory: Health
http://www.directory.google.com/top/health

Search Health and Disabilities and scroll down to disability topic A to Z of interest.

➤ Magellan: Health
  http://www.magellan.excite.com/health

Click on Disabilities and go to subtopics on disabilities.

➤ WebCrawler: Health
  http://www.webcrawler.com/health

Go to the Directory for wide range of information on disability topics of interest.

Disease Control and Prevention

➤ Centers for Disease Control and Prevention
  http://www.cdc.gov
  http://www.cdc.gov/health

U.S. Government agency for information on disease prevention, diagnosis, control and treatment. Provides guidelines to help healthcare professionals and patients.

Provides information on a variety of diseases/disorders/subjects A to Z such as:

- AIDS
- Antibiotic resistance
- Botulism
- Diabetes
- Disease prevention
- Environmental health

- Food borne disease
- Flu vaccine
- Genetics
- Hazardous waste
- Healthy child care
- Health statistics
- Hepatitis
- Hantavirus
- Immunizations
- Injury prevention and control
- Leading causes of death
- Lyme disease
- Measles/mumps/rubella vaccine
- Obesity
- Oral health
- Pollution
- Suicide
- Salmonellosis
- Tobacco
- Toxic chemicals
- Travel health
- Tuberculosis
- Violence
- Water fluoridation

Search site is provided to obtain further information.

Doctor's Guide to Internet
http://www.pslgroup.com

- Current information sites on:
- Diseases and conditions A to Z

• Medical conferences
• Medical news and alerts

Drugs and Medications

➤ Drug Info Net
   http:// www. druginfonet.com

One-stop site for healthcare and drug/medication informational needs. Provides information and links to areas on the Web concerning healthcare and pharmaceutical-related topics. Subscribes to the HON code.

➤ Family Meds.com
   http:// www. familymeds.com

Information on prescription and over the counter drugs. Provides information and clinical recommendations for your health needs. Clinical focus sites include:

  • Diabetes
  • Diseases and conditions
  • Health care
  • Home health
  • Nutrition
  • Personal health
  • Prescription drugs
  • Skin conditions

The Health Clinics site offers information and clinical recommendations for your health needs.
➤ Pharmaceutical Information Network
   http://www.pharminfo.com

Resource for prescription and over the counter drug information and complementary medicines. Disease Info Centers provides information about a particular disease or medical condition by clicking on a topic of interest. A glossary of terms is included along with PharmLinks. A member of the Mediconsult Health Network (http://www.mediconsult.com). Visits to other Health Sites is available as well.

➤ Planet Rx.com
  http://www.planetrx.com

Online pharmacy (drugstore) for prescription and over the counter drugs as well as healthcare information. Sites featured include:

- Alzheimers.com
- Arthritis.com
- Breastcancer.com
- Cholesterol.com
- Depression.com
- Diabetes.com
- Epilepsy.com
- Hepatitis.com
- Weight loss

The interactive tool, "Are you at risk?" helps you improve the state of your health.

➤ Rx List (The Internet Drug Index)
  http://www.rxlist.com

The Internet Drug Index, a Health Central.com Network Site. Provides for keyword search (brands, drug actions, and interactions), the top 200 drugs in the past 5 years, alternative medicine (frequently asked questions and answers, herbs, homeopathics, chinese herbs, ayurvedics), Rx Board (drug specific discussions), Rx List ID (search by imprint codes), search *Taber's Medical Dictionary*, patient education, and about RxList.

➤ Food and Drug Administration (FDA)
  http://www.fda.gov
  http://www.fda.gov/oc/buyonline
  http://www.fda.gov/medwatch

Provides tips, warnings, and advice for consumers buying prescription and other medications on the Internet.

Comprehensive resource on human drugs, foods, biologics, animal drugs, cosmetics, medical devices, radiological health, regulations, toxicology, medical products and Med Watch (reporting and safety information). Provides special information for both patients and health professionals on:

- Consumer product information
- Drug safety and side effects
- FDA drug approval list
- New prescription drug approvals
- Over the counter drug information
- Prescription drug information
- Public health alerts and warning letters
- Reports and publications
- Special projects and programs
- Useful resources

MedWatch, the FDA Medical Products Reporting program, enhances the effectiveness of postmarketing surveillance of medical products as they are used in clinical practice and rapidly identifies significant health hazards associated with a product.

➤ U.S. Pharmacopoeia (USP)
   http://www.usp.org/body.htm

Information about USP, drug standards, drug information, dietary supplements, practitioner reporting and veterinary medicine. Guiding principles for enhancing the likelihood of positive medication use outcomes in geriatric patients is available for review.

➤ Verified Internet Pharmacy Practice Sites
   http://www.nabp.net/vipps/intro.asp

This consumer oriented Web site was established by the FDA in response to illegal Internet drug sales.

Search for online pharmacies that comply with the licensing and inspection requirements of their state and each state to which they dispense pharmaceuticals.

This site warns that: "Buying prescription drugs on the Internet may save you time and perhaps even money. However, buyer beware. Some Web sites may illegally sell prescription drugs without a prescription or sell you such medications if you pass what is regarded as an online consultation (consisting of filling out an electronic questionnaire). It is "legal" for the consumer to buy prescription drugs over the Internet. However, it is "illegal", under Federal and most state law, for anyone to sell prescription drugs without a prescription online or off. Also, it is "illegal" to import prescription drugs into the USA without a prescription. Therefore, if one purchases from an overseas site, your prescription drug package may be seized by customs and your money lost. Reputable Web pharmacies require a faxed copy of your prescription or a phone call from your physician to dispense prescription drugs. Web sites that sell prescription drugs over the Internet may be based in foreign countries. Out of reach of the FDA and US regulations, they may sell substandard, mislabeled, dangerous or abuse potential drugs. Therefor, prudence would dictate that one not buy drugs from these sites even if you have a prescription. Bear in mind that there is no guarantee that you will even receive what you have paid for."

Ear, Nose and Throat Disorders (Otolaryngology)

➤ American Academy of Allergy, Asthma and Immunology
http://www.aaaai.org

Allergic disorders of ear, nose and throat.

➤ American Academy of Audiology
http://www.audiology.org

Hearing disorders.

➤ American Academy of Dermatology
http://www.aad.org

Skin disorders of ear and nose.

➤ American Academy of Facial Plastic and Reconstructive Surgery
http://www.facial_plastic_surgery.org

Plastic and reconstructive surgery of ear, nose and throat.

➤ American Academy of Otolaryngology
http://www.entnet.org
http://www.entnet.org/patient/html

Disorders of nose and throat.

➤ American Academy of Otolaryngic Allergy
   http://www.allergy_ent.org

   Allergic disorders of ear, nose and throat

➤ Colds and Flu
   http://www.4colds4anything.com
   http://www.4flu4anything.com

   Common cold and flu information.

➤ Digestive Health Resource Center
   http://www.gastro.org/public/digestinfo.html

   Disorders of throat/swallowing.

➤ National Institute of Allergy and Infectious Disease
   http://www.niaid.nih.gov

   Allergic and infectious disorders of ear, nose and throat.

➤ National Cancer Institute
   http://www.nci.nih.gov

   Cancer of ear, nose or throat information.

Eating Disorders

➤ American Academy Family Physicians
   http://www.aafp.org

   Eating disorders information can be obtained via search site.

➤ American Medical Association
   http://www.ama-assn.org

Use search site to obtain available information on eating disorders, obesity, etc.

➤ American Psychiatric Association
   http://www.psych.org

Search site provides information on eating disorders.

➤ Center for Disease Control and Prevention
   http://www.cdc.gov

Go to Health Topics A to Z and click on E for Eating Disorders, O for Obesity, etc. to obtain desired information on various eating disorders.

➤ Center for Eating Disorders
   http://www.eatingdisorders.org

Provides information on the diagnosis and treatment of the major eating disorders, what you need to know about eating disorders, joining a discussion group, questions and answers, latest news and top ten links on the subject

➤ Endocrine Society
   http://www.endo-society.org

Information on various eating disorders and body weight issues.

➤ Take Off Pounds Sensibly

http://www.tops.org

Dedicated to helping people take and keep off pounds sensibly. Provides for a chapter locator near you, general information, frequently asked questions and answers and links.

Endocrine Disorders

➤ Endocrine Society
  http://www.endo-society.org

Valuable resource for information on a variety of endocrine disorders such as:

- Benign prostatic hypertropy
- Birth defects
- Breast cancer
- Body weight issues
- Cushing's syndrome
- Diabetes
- Eating disorders
- Endometriosis
- Environmental estrogens
- Erectile dysfunction
- Female infertility
- Genetics
- High cholesterol
- Hirsutism
- Male infertility
- Menopause
- Premature birth
- Premenstrual syndrome

- Prostate cancer
- Respiratory distress syndrome
- Short stature
- Stress related disease
- Thyroid disorders
- Turner's syndrome

➢ National Institute of Diabetes and Digestive and Kidney Diseases
    http://www.niddk.nih.gov

Premier source for information on diabetes. Also see Diabetes Mellitus Health Category #23 for further information on the subject.

➢ Thyroid Foundation of America
    http://www.tsh.org.main.html

Provides patients with educational brochures about thyroid disorders, books which explain how your thyroid works, newsletter with articles by thyroid experts, referrals to thyroid specialist in your area, and other publications and web resources/sites.

Environmental Health and Safety

➢ American College of Occupational and Environmental Medicine
    http://www.acoem.org

Provides courses, conferences, newsletters, *Journal of Occupational and Environmental Medicine* online, and numerous other services. Links to other occupational and environmental medicine resources are available.

➢ Centers for Disease Control and Prevention
    http://www.cdc.gov/health

Go to Health Topics A to Z and click on Environmental Health and Safety for information on environment-related disorders, their prevention, and treatment.

➤ Occupational Safety and Health Administration
   http://www.osha.gov/safelinks.html

All about occupational health and safety information from the U.S. Government.

➤ National Institute of Environmental Health Sciences
   http://www.nichs.nih.gov

Leading Federal effort on environmental health and safety.

Epilepsy

➤ American Epilepsy Society
   http://www.aesnet.org

Research and education information for professionals, patients and consumers. Dedicated to the prevention and treatment of epilepsy. *Epilepsia* provides electronic access to full text articles. Provides information on drug alerts, new developments in the field, treatments and web links.

➤ Epilepsy.com
   http://www.epilepsy.com

Powered by Planet Rx.com. Provides numerous special topic sites for epilepsy information. You may use the search site to obtain further information of interest.

➤ National Institute of Neurological Disorders and Stroke
http://www.ninds.nih.gov

Leading Federal effort regarding epilepsy. Research, diagnosis, treatment and links. Search site provided for information of interest regarding epilepsy.

Eye Disorders

➤ American Academy of Ophthalmology
http://www.eyenet.org

Eye anatomy, health, disease, conditions and consumer advocacy. Featured topic sites include:

- Cataracts
- Diabetic retinopathy
- Glaucoma
- Macular degeneration
- Refractive eye surgery

➤ American Foundation for the Blind
http://www.afb.org

Mission is to enable people who are blind or visually impaired to achieve equality of access and opportunity. Blindness information, resources, reports, fact sheets and more are available.

➤ International Society of Refractive Surgery
http://www.isrs.org

Information on the art and science of refractive surgery including sites for:
- locate a doctor
- search for information on refractive eye surgery.

➤ Glaucoma Research Foundation
   http://www.glaucoma.org/glaucoma.html

Glaucoma, diagnosis, treatment and related resources information.

➤ Lighthouse International
   http://www.lighthouse.org

Resource for major causes and what can be done to improve low vision. Eye care tips, eye conditions, vision health and advocacy sites are provided.

➤ National Eye Institute
   http://www.nei.nih.gov

Leading U.S. Government effort regarding eye disorders information for researchers, health care professionals, educators and the public and patients. Use search site for eye disorder information of interest. A low vision education program, clinical studies database of ongoing and completed studies and a national eye health education program are available.

Family Medical and Health

➤ American Academy of Family Physicians
   http:// www.aafp.org
Family health resource. Provides for online search of family health and wellness issues, diseases and conditions, recommendations regarding periodic health examinations and recommended immunization schedules.

Fitness, Diet, and Exercise

➤ American Heart Association
  http://www.americanheart.org
  http://www.americanheart.org/dietaryguidelines/index.html

Health, fitness, diets, and exercise information to prevent heart disease, stroke and lower cholesterol are available. See Dietary Guidelines: Revision 2000 official recommendations.

➤ American Hiking Society
  http://www.americanhiking.org

National organization dedicated to serving hikers and protecting the nation's hiking trails. Hikers Info Center trail conservation and policy, events and volunteer opportunities, Alliance of Hiking Organizations, news and resources, Hiker's Emporium, Join American Hiking, and Inside American Hiking are some of the resources provided.

➤ eFit (Online Health and Fitness Network)
  http://www.efit.com
  http://www.efit.com/basics

What you need to know to get started on your favorite activity and fitness plan. Provides key information on:

- Cardio basic/fitness
- Cooking and nutrition
- Cycling
- Diet and weight loss
- Kids fitness
- Hips/abs/thighs

- Running
- Snow sports
- Strength training
- Teen's health/fitness
- Walking and hiking
- Yoga/mind/body

Features following health living tools:

- Activity/calorie calculator
- Body mass index
- Fitness calculator
- Food/nutrition search
- Gym locator
- Health and medical dictionary
- Healthy living portal
- Healthy restaurant locator

Diet, exercise, and custom programs are available.

➤ Fitness Center
   http://www.justmove.org/home.cfm

Keep track of your fitness progress online and sign up for your own personal trainer. Obtain the latest health, heart and fitness information as well as frequently asked questions and answers and health facts. Find out what fitness category you fall into. Compare yourself to the rest of the USA using their national fitness database. Connect with others around the world with fitness related interests via their forum. Local, regional and national fitness events are featured. Use their search site to obtain information you are looking for.

➤ FitnessLink
   http://www.fitnesslink.com

Athletic adventures, exercise encyclopedia, virtual gym, home gym, nutrition and diet, mind and body, men's locker room, women's locker room, pro's center, total wellness, juice bar and quick search tools are some of the sites featured.

➤ Fitness at Women.com
   http://www.women.com/fitness

Weight loss, diet, nutrition, exercise, weight training, lose weight, aerobics, calories and tools and advice for your fitness and weight loss needs information sites are featured.

➤ Forest Service
   http://www.fs.fed.us

Recreation, sports, hiking, walking, enjoyment of outdoors, and beauty of nature in U.S. National Forests.

➤ Global Fitness and Health
   http://www.global_fitness.com

Extensive fitness and health information.

➤ Great Outdoors Recreation Pages
   http://www.gorp.com

All about recreation, sports, hiking, walking, and enjoyment of outdoors provided.

➤ National Park Service
   http://www.nps.gov

Recreation, sports, hiking, walking and enjoyment of outdoors and beauty of nature opportunities in U.S. National Parks.

➤ Outdoors.org
   http://www.outdoors.org

Features a wide variety of outdoor activities and places to improve fitness and enhance weight control and health.

➤ Recreation.Gov
   http://www.recreation.gov

Recreational opportunities on US federal lands. Allows one to search for recreation sites by state, agency or recreational activity.

➤ Shape Up America
   http://www.shapeup.org

Provides the latest comprehensive information about safe weight management and physical fitness.

➤ Weights.Net
   http://www.weightsnet.com

Resource for people who workout with weights for body building, fitness, power lifting, sports and more.

Genetic Disorders

➤ American College of Medical Genetics

http://www.faseb.org/genetics/acmg/acmgmenu.htm

Provides information on genetic susceptibility to disease, and standards and guidelines for clinical genetics laboratories. Official journal, *Genetics in Medicine*, is available online.

➢ National Human Genome Research Institute
http://www.nhgri.nih.gov/index.html

Information on the human genome project. Serves as a center for inherited disease research, as well as ethical, legal and social implications, policy and public affairs. Provides genomic and genetic resources, workshops and conferences, glossary of genetic terms, news, and search site to obtain information on genetic topics of interest.

Harvard Medical Center

➢ Harvard Medical Web
http://www.med.harvard.edu

With nearly 8,000 faculty and 17 affiliated health facilities, the Harvard Medical Community research, health information, and patient care are among the best available anywhere in the world. Search health topics of interest on the sites provided.

➢ Harvard Health Publications
http://www.health.harvard.edu/newsletters

Obtain information on a spectrum of health topics written about in the last decade via the subject index on this web site which lists over 2,000 articles from all five Harvard Health Newsletters. Selected articles may be reviewed or downloaded for a small fee. Other articles are available from back issues which can be ordered through the web site, or by phone, fax or mail. Go to the searchable index for information of interest.

Headache

➤ American Academy of Neurology
   http://www.aan.com

   Headache guidelines and neurology online. Use search site provided to obtain any headache information of interest.

➤ Headache.com
   http://www.headache.com.au

   Discusses various types of headaches and provides statistics, causes and treatments.

➤ Headache.net
   http://www.headache.net/html/netscape.html

   Specializes in the diagnosis, treatment and patient education of various kinds of headaches.

➤ National Headache Foundation
   http://www.headaches.org

   Educational and support services to headache and migraine sufferers through newsletters, support groups, counseling, referrals, conferences and presentations.

➤ National Institute of Neurological Disorders and Stroke
   http://www.ninds.nih.gov

Leading U.S. Government effort regarding headache information, research, diagnosis and treatment. Use search site provided to obtain headache information of interest.

Healthcare Research and Quality

➤ Agency for Healthcare Research and Quality
   http://www.ahrq.gov
   http://www.ahrq.gov/consumer/20tips.htm
   http://www.ahrq.gov/qual/errors.htm

Leading Federal effort regarding information on healthcare information research and quality. Featured topics include:

- Children's health
- Clinical practice guidelines
- Consumer assessment of health plans
- Evidence based practice
- Health costs and utilization
- Healthfinder.gov
- Health guides
- HIV cost and use
- Long term care
- Managed care
- Medical Errors
- Medical expenditure
- Outcomes
- Preventive services
- Prescriptions
- Primary care
- Quality measurement

- Specific health conditions
- Surgery
- Technology assessment
- 20 tips
- User liaison program
- Women's health

Search sites provided for further information by topic and category.

Health Insurance

➢ American Medical Association
   http://www.ama-assn.org

Go to Consumer Health and then to Choosing Your Health Plan.

➢ Symphony Group
   http://www.thesymphonygroup.com

Healthcare professionals offering you health insurance information and resources. This site answers questions you may have about health insurance and you may submit a question of interest on health insurance.

Hearing

➢ American Academy of Audiology
   http://www.audiology.org

Information on hearing for consumers and professionals including news, an audiologist finder and links.

➢ American Academy of Otolaryngology

http://www.entnet.org
http://www.entnet.org/patient.html

Information on disorders of the ear, nose, and throat as well as related conditions of the head, neck and hearing. Sites for diseases, conditions, topics, patient information, research and web links are available. Search is provided for information on hearing disorder topics of interest.

➤ American Academy of Otolaryngic Allergy
   http://www.allergy_ent.org

In formation on allergic conditions which may affect hearing.

➤ National Institute on Deafness and Other Communication Disorders
   http://www.nih.gov/nidcd

Leading U.S. Government effort regarding information on deafness and hearing problems and other communication disorders.

Home Health

➤ American Academy of Family Physicians
   http://www.aafp.org

Search for home health information.

➤ American Medical Association
   http://www.ama-assn.org

Search for home health information.

➤ Google Web Directory: Health

http://www.directory google.com/top/health

Go to Home Health for information.

➢ Lycos Directory: Health
http://www.lycos.com/health

Click on Health and go to Home Health site.

➢ Netscape: Health
http://www.health.netscape.com/health.main.tmpl

Go to information on Health Search Categories and click on Home Health.

Hospitals

➢ Association of American Medical Colleges
http://www.aamc.org
➢ Internet Hospital Directory
http://www.dis.dial.pipex.com/r.bowyer/hospital.html
➢ Internet Medical School Directory
http://www.ds.dial.pipex.com/r.bowyer/med_schl.htm
➢ Medline (National Library of Medicine)
http://www.nlm.nih.gov/medline
➢ Medlineplus (National Library of Medicine)
http://www.nlm.nih.gov/medlineplus

Above five references provide information on university, medical college, and teaching hospitals throughout the USA and internationally as well as the medical information they offer.

Human Anatomy

➤ American Medical Association
http://www.ama-assn.org

Go to Consumer Health Site and click on Human Atlas.

➤ Achoo Gateway to Healthcare (Human Health and Disease Directory)
http://www.achoo.com/directory/hhd/disease.asp

Go to human anatomy site.

➤ Infoseek: Health and Wellness
http://infoseek.go.com
http://www.infoseek.go.com/webdir/health

Go to Medical Reference Topics and click on human anatomy.

Hypertension

➤ American College of Cardiology
http://www.acc.org

Search site provides information on hypertension.

➤ American Heart Association
http://www.americanheart.org

Go to Heart and Stroke A to Z and click on hypertension to obtain information.

➤ LifeClinic.com

http://www.lifeclinic.com

Features medical products used by physicians and consumers to monitor blood pressure. Provides a unique online resource for health information and empowers people to take control of their health by monitoring their blood pressure, cholesterol, pulse and weight, free of charge, and with a high level of convenience, accuracy and security.

➤ National Heart, Lung and Blood Institute (NHLBI)
  http://www.nhlbi.nih.gov

Use NHLBI search site to obtain information of interest on hypertension.

Hypnosis

➤ American Medical Association
  http://www.ama-assn.org

Use search site for information on hypnosis.

➤ American Psychiatric Association
  http://www.psych.org/main.html

Use search site for information on hypnosis.

➤ Society for Clinical and Experimental Hypnosis
  http://www.sunsite.utk.edu/IJCEH/scehframe.htm

Organization dedicated to research and application of hypnosis in the clinical setting. *International Journal of Clinical and Experimental Hypnosis* provides a special issue on empirical validation of hypnosis clinical interventions. You may consult with an expert in the field via this site.

Industrial and Occupation Health

➤ Achoo Gateway to Healthcare (Human Health and Disease Directory)
http://www.achoo.com/directory/hhd/disease.asp

Under Diseases and Conditions, click on Injury or Occupational Disease.

➤ American College of Occupational and Environmental Medicine
http://www.acoem.org

Provides courses and conferences, newsletters, *Journal of Occupational and Environmental Medicine* online, and numerous other services and general information, what's new, position statements, guidelines, and links to other related resources.

➤ American Industrial Hygiene Association
http://www.aiha.org

Features sites for consumer information, news, Academy of Industrial Hygiene, conferences and meetings, publications and periodicals.

➤ Centers for Disease Control and Prevention
http://www.cdc.gov/health

Go to Health Topics A to Z and click on Occupational Health for information on industrial hygiene/occupational health topics of interest use CDC search site for additional information.

➤ National Institute of Environmental Health Sciences
http://www.niehs.nih.gov

Premier Federal information site on industrial/occupational health.

Infectious Disease

➤ Centers for Disease Control and Prevention
   http://www.cdc.gov/health

   Premier Federal resource on infectious disease, statistics, diagnosis and treatment. Use CDC search site to obtain infectious disease information of interest.

➤ Google Web Directory: Health
   http://www.google.com/top/health

   Go to Conditions and Disease Categories and click on Infectious Disease.

➤ National Institute of Allergy and Infectious Diseases
   http://www.niaid.nih.gov

   Go to information sites on Infectious Diseases and Vaccines. Use search site provided to obtain further information on infectious diseases.

Internal Medicine

➤ American College of Physicians/American Society of Internal Medicine
   (ACP/ASIM)
   http://www.acponline.org
   http://www.asim.org

   Provides information on internal medical disorders. Features sites for:

   • Annals of Internal Medicine online
   • Diseases, conditions, and topic search

- For Internists (clinical info, computers, practice tips, publications, etc.)
- Interact with ACP/ASIM (discussion groups, links, etc.)
- News
- Publications (reports)
- Web sites for internists

➤ Society of General Internal Medicine
http://www.sgim.org

General internal medicine information sites on:

- Anticoagulation and thromboembolism
- Clinical examination research
- Health policy
- Hospitalists
- International health
- Medical consultation
- Medical problems in pregnancy and obstetric medicine
- Minorities in medicine
- Physicians against violence
- Primary care
- Research
- Social responsibility
- Substance abuse
- Violence
- Women's caucus

➤ Medicine and Medical Specialties
http://www.directory.google.com/top/health/medicine/medical_specialties

Journal of the American Medical Association
http://www.jama.ama-assn.org

Features medical news, articles, and editorials on health, wellness, healthcare and internal medicine topics, diseases and conditions.

Kidney Disease

➤ American College of Physicians
   http://www.acponline.org

Use search site for information on kidney diseases and topics of interest about kidney disease.

➤ National Institute of Diabetes and Digestive and Kidney Diseases
   http://www.niddk.nih.gov

Leading Federal effort providing information on all aspects of kidney disease/ disorders, diagnosis, treatment and statistics. Use search site provided to obtain additional information on kidney disorders.

➤ National Kidney Foundation
   http://www.kidney.org

Information on organ and tissue donors and recipients, healthcare professionals in the field, patient information, and meetings, events, and news. Use search site provided to obtain information on kidney disorders.

Lancet
http://www.thelancet.com

Premier international journal of medical science and practice. Search The Lancet database for diseases, conditions, and topics of interest.

Leukemia and Lymphoma

➤ Leukemia and Lymphoma Society
   http://www.leukemia-lymphoma.org

Leukemia and lymphoma information. See National Cancer Institute Web site (http://www.nci.nih.gov) for additional information on leukemias and lymphomas.

Medical Colleges/Schools

➤ Association of American Medical Colleges
   http://www.aamc.org

List of member medical colleges in the U.S. and Canada that provide a wealth of information on diseases, conditions, and topics of interest.

➤ Internet Medical School Directory
   http://www.ds.dial.pipex.com/r.bowyer/med_schl.htm

Medical colleges and health information they may offer.

Medical Dictionary and Medical Encyclopedia

Available via the following web sites:

➤ American Medical Association
   http://www.ama-assn.org
➤ Healthfinder

http://www.healthfinder.gov
➤ Mayo Clinic Health Oasis
   http:// www.mayohealth.org
➤ Medline
   http://www.nlm.nih.gov/medline
➤ Medline Plus
   http:// www. nlm.nih.gov/medlineplus
➤ National Network of Libraries of Medicine
   http://www.nnlm.nlm.nih.gov/psr

Meditation

➤ Doctor's Guide to the Internet (Mediation)
   http://www.pslgroup.com/meditation

➤ Learning Meditation Home Page
   http://www.learningmeditation.com

Conscious relaxation and stress reduction through mediation. Real Audio mediations allows you to listen, relax and achieve inner peace right on the web. Favorite web links are provided.

➤ Meditation.com
   http://www.meditation.com

You may click onto the follow mediation sites:
   • Common as Rain offers relaxing guidance. Lectures are also available.
   • How to Meditate may be a useful aid to calmness, clarity of mind and ultimately inner peace.
   • Meditation Made Easy teaches how to eliminate stress and anxiety from the BTS International Medication Institute.

• Power of Meditation and Prayer provides an expansive view of the nature of the process from several perspectives.

Several meditation center sites are available for further information.

➤ Medlineplus (Meditation)
  http://www.nlm.nih.gov/medlineplus/meditation

Provides mediation information available via National Library of Medicine.

➤ Yahoo.com
  http://www.health.yahoo.com

Use Yahoo search site to obtain information on meditation.

Medline
http://www.nlm.nih.gov/medline

Medlineplus
http://www.nlm.nih.gov/medlineplus

Above two Web resources/sites provide comprehensive health information from over 10 million citations worldwide on:

- Diseases and conditions A to Z
- Diagnosis and treatment
- Hospitals
- Libraries
- Medical dictionary
- Medical encyclopedia
- Medications
- Organizations
- Publications and news
- Research
- Search by health topic categories offered
- Search Medline or Medlineplus
- Selected new sites and links

Men's Health

➢ American Academy of Family Physicians
   http://www.aafp.org
➢ American Medical Association
   http://www.ama-assn.org
➢ Intelihealth
   http://www intelihealth.com
➢ Mayo Clinic Health Oasis
   http://www.mayohealth.org

All four resources and Web sites provide extensive information about men's health, diet, exercise, fitness and more.

Mental Health

➢ Academy of Psychosomatic Medicine
   http://www.apm.org

Mind body medicine information, clinical liaison psychiatry information regarding mental disorders superimposed on medical conditions.

➤ American Academy of Child and Adolescent Psychiatry
  http://www.aacap.org

  Features sites on:

  • Advocacy groups
  • Clinical practice
  • Facts for families
  • Hot topics
  • Journals
  • Legislation
  • Other resources
  • Regional organizations
  • Research
  • Resource links to other organizations
  • Search for further information
  • What's new

➤ American Academy of Clinical Psychiatrists
  http://www.aacp.com

Consumer information on mind/body connection and resources for individuals about when and how to seek help for problems with work, family and relationships.

➤ American Psychiatric Association (APA)
  http://www.psych.org/main/html

Information on:

- APA online clinical resources
- Diagnosis and treatment of mental and emotional illnesses and substance abuse disorders
- Dictionaries
- Frequently asked questions and answers
- Journals
- Major and minor focus areas, diseases, and conditions
- Special groups
- What's new

➤ American Psychoanalytic Association
  http://www.apsa.org

Information on psychoanalysis. Journal online and links to other resources.

➤ American Psychological Association
  http://www.helping.apa.org

Psychology and counseling information.

➤ American Psychosomatic Society
  http://www.psychosomatic.org

Mind and body interrelationships in health and disease.

➤ Cyber Psych Link
  http://www.cyber_psych.org

Information and links regarding psychology and behavorial medicine. List of services and databases.

➢ Depression.comh
   htttp://www.depression.com

News and information about depression and its treatment, with individual sections devoted to specific types of depression, symptoms and treatment.

➢ Internet Mental Health
   http://www.mentalhealth.com

Encyclopedia of information on mental illnesses, treatments, medications, research, and findings. Covers over 50 of the most common mental disorders, over 70 of the most common psychiatric drugs, latest research findings for each mental illness and medication and links to other mental health sites. Translations into a number of languages are available.

➢ Mental Health Net
   http://www.mentalhelp.net

One of the oldest and largest online mental health guides. Features information on:

• Diagnostic criteria assessment
• Disorders and treatment
• Find clinics and treatment facilities
• Find a therapist
• Find an online therapist
• Forums and chat groups
• Glossary of mental health terms
• Managed care glossary
• Medication information
• Research studies
• Search MHN and Medline databases for additional information

➤ National Alliance for the Mentally Ill
   http://www.nami.org

Mental disorders/illnesses, medications, research, links, help line and search site for further information.

➤ National Institute on Drug Abuse
   http://www.nida.nih.gov

Leading Federal effort on drug abuse, what's new, publications, other links. Search site provided for additional information.

➤ National Institute of Mental Health
   http://www.nimh.nih.gov

Leading U.S. Government effort on mental health disorders and issues for the public, patients, practitioners and researchers. Current mental health topics are featured. Search site provided to obtain further information.

➤ National Mental Health Association
   http://www. nmha.org

Provides useful information on mental health.

Mental Retardation

➤ American Association on Mental Retardation
   http://www.aamr.org/index
➤ Association for Retarded Citizens (The Arc of the United States)
   http://www.thearc.org
➤ National organization regarding mental retardation and related
   disabilities and their families. News, services, state and local chapters,

position statements, frequently asked questions and answers, publications, videos and related links are provided.

➤ National Association for Down Syndrome Society
   http://www.nads.org
➤ National Down Syndrome Society
   http://www.ndss.org
➤ National Institute of Child Health and Human Development
   http://www.nichd.nih.gov

Above five organizations provide information regarding mental retardation, related disabilities, news, services, state and local chapters, frequently asked questions and answers, publications, and related links.

Merck Manual
http://www.merck.com/pubs/mmanual

Information on a large number of health topics. One of the world's most widely used medical texts available in 14 languages. Information is provided in 23 categories in 308 chapters as follows:

• Cardiovascular
• Clinical pharmacology
• Dental and Oral
• Dermatologic
• Ear/nose/throat
• Endocrine
• Gastrointestinal
• Gynecology and obstetrics
• Hematology and oncology
• Hepatic and bilary
• Immunology and allergy
• Infectious

- Musculoskeletal and connective tissue
- Neurology
- Nutritional
- Ophthalmologic
- Pediatrics
- Physical agents
- Poisoning
- Psychiatric
- Pulmonary
- Special subjects

Use search site to obtain additional information of interest.

Musculoskeletal and Orthopedic Disorders

➤ American Academy of Orthopedic Surgeons
  http://www.aaos.org

Educational programs for orthopedic surgeons, allied health professionals, patients and the public. Sites for finding an orthopedic surgeon and outcomes/guidelines are available along with other links. You may search Medline or the AAOS site for further information on musculoskeletal/orthopedic disorders of interest.

➤ American Orthopedic Foot and Ankle Society (AAFAS)
  http://www.aofas.org

Foot and ankle disorders/treatment with member locator service. Provides AAFAS guides to *Foot Fitness For Life* as well as *Your Feet Young and Healthy*

➤ American Podiatric Medical Association

http://www.apma.org

Features foot disorders topics such as:

- Aerobics
- Aging feet
- Arthritis
- Athlete's foot
- Children' feet
- Diabetes and the feet
- Flying
- Foot and ankle injuries
- Foot health
- Foot surgery
- Footwear
- Fungal nails
- General foot fitness
- Heel pain
- Nail problems
- On-the-job foot health
- Orthotics
- Sports and the feet/ankle
- Rear foot surgery
- Warts, plantar
- Women's feet problems

➤ Back Pain Resource Center
   http://www.backpainreliefonline.com

Information on back pain causes/relief.

➤ Medlineplus (Arthritis)

http://www.nlm.nih.gov/medlineplus/arthritis.html

Information on all forms of arthritis and related categories: bones, joints, muscles, senior health, gout/pseudogout, juvenile rheumatoid arthritis, osteoarthritis, rheumatoid arthritis and more.

➢ Muscular Dystropy Association
   http://www. mdausa.org

Muscular dystropy and other neuromuscular disorders and other resources.

➢ National Chronic Fatigue and Fibromyalgia Association
   http://www.cfidsfoundation.org

Latest information on chronic fatigue syndrome and fibromyalgia plus other resources.

➢ National Institute of Arthritis and Musculoskeletal and Skin Diseases
   http://www.nih.gov/niams
   http://www.nih.gov/niams/healthinfo

Information on normal structure and function of joints, muscles, and bones. Also covers musculoskeletal diseases and conditions including heritable disorders of bone and cartilage, inherited and inflammatory muscle diseases, sports injuries and rehabilitation medicine, and cancer. Search site allows you to obtain further information on musculoskeletal/orthopedic disorders. Additional information, scientific resources, clinical studies and reports also are available.

➢ National Osteoporosis Foundation
   http://www.nof.org

Patient information on osteoporosis, prevention, treatment and advocacy. Physician's Guide to Osteoporosis Prevention and Treatment developed in collaboration with 10 multidisciplinary medical organizations gives practicing physicians and patients specific recommendations for managing and preventing osteoporosis. Find a doctor or specialist service is provided.

➤ Spine Health (Back Pain)
  http://www.spine_health.com

A comprehensive resource for:

- Anatomy and back pain
- Common causes and diagnoses back pain
- Conservative treatments
- Degenerative disc disease
- Diagnostic tests/studies
- Disc herniation
- Fibromyalgia
- Injection sites for pain relief
- Low back/neck pain
- Osteoarthritis
- Osteoporosis
- Physical therapy
- Surgical treatments

Additional sites featured provide information on:
- Degenerative disc disease and non-surgical treatment options
- Effective coping strategies for chronic pain
- Find a specialist
- How a physical therapist can help with exercise
- Send a question to a specialist

- Today's healthy back tip
- Treatment options for lumbar disc herniation
- What to expect at your first chiropractic visit
- When to see a surgeon for lower back pain

National Institutes of Health Institutes and Centers
http://www.nih.gov.icd

National Institutes of Health is comprised of 25 separate Institutes and Centers and is one of 8 health agencies of the U.S. Department of Health and Human Services. Click on appropriate Institute or Center to obtain information of interest.

Institutes and Centers are:
- National Cancer Institute
- National Center for Complementary and Alternative Medicine
- National Center for Information Technology
- National Center for Research Resources
- National Center for Scientific Review
- National Center on Sleep Disorders
- National Eye Institute
- National Heart, Lung and Blood Institute
- National Human Genome Research Institute
- National Institute on Aging
- National Institute on Alcohol Abuse and Alcoholism
- National Institute of Allergy and Infectious Diseases
- National Institute on Arthritis, Musculoskeletal and Skin Diseases
- National Institute of Child Health and Human Development
- National Institute of Deafness and Other Communication Disorders
- National Institute of Dental and Craniofacial Research
- National Institute of Diabetes, Digestive and Kidney Diseases
- National Institute on Drug Abuse

• National Institute of Environmental Health Sciences
• National Institutes of General Medical Sciences
• National Institute of Mental Health
• National Institute of Neurological Disorders and Stroke
• National Institute of Nursing Research
• National Institutes of Health John E. Fogarty International Center
• National Institutes of Health Warren Grant Magnuson Clinical Center

See Chapters IV and VI Web Sites for each center or institute. Go to nih.gov/health for further health information.

National Library of Medicine
http://www.nlm.nih.gov

World's largest medical library. Health information available via Medline, Medlineplus, and other resources. Provides access to Clinical Trials.gov for information for patients about clinical research studies that may be available for treatment.

Neurological Disorders

➤ American Academy of Neurology
   http://www.aan.com

Features neurology online, headache guidelines and a site to search for further neurological disorders information of interest.

➤ American Academy of Neurological and Orthopedic Surgeons
   http://www.aanos.org

AANOS journal, patient information and links to other sites.

➤ American Academy of Neurological Surgeons
http://www.neurosurgery.org/aans

Neurosurgery on call, health resources and other information

➤ American Epilepsy Society
http://www.aesnet.org

Information on epilepsy. See Chapter V: Health Categories, Disease, Resources, and Web Sites for further epilepsy information.

➤ National Institute of Neurological Disorders and Stroke
http://www.ninds.nih.gov

Leading Federal effort on neurological disorders and stroke. Provides information for the public, patients, clinicians and scientists. Obtain further information via their search site. Health Publications A to Z are available.

➤ National Multiple Sclerosis Society
http://www.nmss.org

Latest multiple sclerosis information and news provided. Local resources and other information are available.

➤ National Parkinson Foundation
http://www.parkinson.org

Parkinson's Disease information for patients and healthcare providers.

New England Journal of Medicine
http://www.nejm.org

Abstracts of articles available. Paid subscription required for full-text articles. Search past issues for information on a wide variety of health topics.

Nuclear Medicine
http://www.snm.org

Relevant information on frequently asked questions and answers and what patients should know about what is nuclear medicine and its procedures. Features imaging information on:

- Bone
- Brain
- Breast
- Colorectal
- Heart
- Links to other sites
- Liver and hepatobilary
- Ovaries
- Prostate
- Renal

Also included is a site for radioiodine imaging and treatment of thyroid disorders.

You may obtain further information on nuclear medicine topics of interest via the SNM search site.

Nutrition, Food and Health

➤ American College of Nutrition
    http://www am_coll_nutr.org

Relevant information on nutrition. *Journal of the American College of Nutrition* online.

➤ American Dietetic Association
   http://www.eatright.org

Information on dietary balance, food variety and moderation, and eating right the healthy way. Access the National Center for Nutrition and Dietetics for sound nutrition information resources and registered dieticians. Features sites on:

- Find a dietician
- Food safety
- Gateway to related sites
- Government affairs
- Marketplace
- News
- Nutrition resources
- Publications

➤ American Heart Association (Dietary Guidelines: Revision 2000)
   http://www.americanheart.org/dietaryguidelines/index.htm

Dietary Guidelines Revision 2000 is designed to help most Americans prevent heart disease, hypertension and stroke. Obesity prevention is one of its top priorities. Detailed dietary information is available for patients who already have heart disease or diabetes, or who have to control their level of cholesterol and/or triglycerides in their blood.

➤ American Society for Clinical Nutrition
   http://www.faseb.org/ascn

An array of information on clinical nutrition. *American Journal Clinical Nutrition* online.

➢ Center for Nutrition Policy and Promotion (US Department of Agriculture)
 http://www.usda.gov/cnpp

Provides relevant information on:

- Breakfast and learning in children
- Childhood obesity
- Dietary behavior: Why we choose the foods we eat
- Dietary guidelines for Americans
- Family economics and nutrition review
- Food guide pyramid
- The great nutrition debate
- Interactive healthy eating index and check you overall diet quality
- Nutrient content of the US food supply
- Nutrition guidelines for Americans
- Nutrition insights
- Recipes and tips for healthy, thrifty meals

Links to:

- Economic research service (food assistance and nutrition research program)
- Food nutrition information service
- Food surveys research group
- Nutrient data laboratory
- Team nutrition
- USDA program missions

➤ Cyber Diet
   http://www.cyberdiet.com

Provides information on a healthy lifestyle, diet, nutrition and weight loss. Features sites for:
- Assessment : assessment tools, body fat distribution, body mass index, risk assessment and waist to hip ratio
- Diet and nutrition: daily food planner, dining out, diet detective, eating right, fast food quest, food facts, good food nutrition bytes, recipe index, and recipe makeovers
- Exercise and fitness: activity calculator, charity events, exercise tips, health club, target heart rate
- Resource center: about cancer, arthritis, ask the experts, asthma and allergy, depression and diet, digestive disorders, every woman, healthy heart, HIV and AIDS, pregnancy and infertility, treating diabetes, and weight loss
- Support and motivation: diet, discussion groups, help desk, meditation room, newsletter, preservers, success

Features daily food planner, good food, good ways, risk assessment, get started with weight loss and express menus.

➤ Food and Health Communications
   http://www.foodandhealth.com

Publisher of nutrition education resources and *Communicating Health Newsletter*. Features sites for:

- Food ingredients
- Foods to prevent disease
- Free newsletter
- Resources for all your nutrition education needs

• Weight loss

➤ Food Safety.Gov
   http://www.foodsafety.gov

   Gateway to government food safety information. Features sites on:

   • Consumer advice
   • Federal and state government agencies
   • Foodborne pathogens
   • Frequently asked questions and answers
   • Kids, teens, and education
   • Natural food safety initiatives
   • News
   • Report illness and product complaint
   • Safety alert
   • Search for food safety information of interest
   • Videos

➤ Interactive Healthy Eating Index
   http://www.usda.gov.cnpp

   Healthy eating guide.

➤ International Food and Information Council
   http://ww.ifcinfo.health.org

   Nutritional information.

➤ Tufts University Nutritional Navigator
   http://www.navigator.tufts.edu

Leading center on nutrition information. Sites for:

- Educators
- Focus on nutrition
- General nutrition
- Hot topics
- Journalists
- Health professionals
- Kids
- Parents
- Special dietary needs
- What's new
- Women

➢ US Department of Agriculture (Nutrient Data Laboratory)
http://www.nal.usda.gov/fnic/foodcomp

Food nutrient composition data. Search for food nutrition values in the USDA Nutrient Database. Research food composition and resource links provided. Frequently asked questions and answers and a glossary of terms as well as selected reports on food topics of interest
➢

Vegetarian Resource Group
http://www.vrg.org

Information on vegetarian diets, nutrition, way of life and benefits.

Obesity and Weight Control

See Health Categories regarding Nutrition, Food, and Health as well as Fitness, Diet, and Exercise for appropriate resources and web sites for information on obesity/ overweight and their prevention and treatment.

Occupational Health and Safety (OSHA)

➤ American College of Occupational and Environmental Medicine
http:www.acoem.org

Courses, conferences, newsletters, *Journal of Occupational and Environmental Medicine* online, links to other OEM resources and services.

➤ Centers for Disease Control and Prevention
http://www.cdc.gov/health

Go to Health Topics A to Z and click on to Occupational Health and Safety information of interest.

➤ Med Explorer
http://www.medexplorer.com

Go to Health Safety site for information on Fire Prevention/Safety, Hygiene, Infection control, Injury prevention and other occupational health information.

➤ National Institute of Environmental Health Sciences➤
http://www.niehs.nih.gov

Key US Government resource regarding occupational health and safety.

➤ Occupational Safety and Health Administration (US Department of Labor) http://www.osha.gov/safelinks.html

OSHA provides numerous occupational safety and health Internet sites that may be helpful and informative.

Orthopedic Disorders

See Musculoskeletal Disorders for disorders and web sites.

Otolaryngology Disorders (Ear, Nose and Throat)

See Ear, Nose and Throat Disorders for disorders and web sites.

Pain

➤ American Academy of Pain Medicine
  http://www.painmed.org

  Extensive pain information resource.

➤ American Academy of Head, Neck and Facial Pain
  http://www.aanhfp.org

  Information on TMJ (temporal mandibular joint) syndrome, dental health, and headaches and dental health.

➤ American Pain Society
  http://www.ampainsoc.org

  Serves people in pain by advancing research, education, treatment and professional practice. Evidence based guidelines for pain management, pain facilities, publications, advocacy and other resources are available.

➤ Pain.com
  http://www.pain.com

  Features pain information on:

- Cancer
- Chatroom
- Clinics
- Interview with experts
- Management, updates, intervention
- Meetings
- Migraine
- News
- Online journal
- Other headaches
- Regional anesthesia treatment
- Resources
- Standards

Parkinson's Disease

➤ American Parkinson's Disease Association
http://www.adaparkinson.com

General information about Parkinson's Disease.

➤ National Parkinson Foundation
http://www.parkinson.org

A world-wide organization providing sites for information on:

- Affiliate chapters
- Ask Dr. Lieberman, Medical Director
- Caregiver's information web site
- Centers of excellence
- Clinical studies
- Conferences and symposia

- Get to know NPF
- Helpful tests
- Helpful resources
- Interaction server and talk with other parkinsonians
- News today and events
- Other links
- Parkinson facts
- Parkinson surgery web site
- Search for further information of interest

Pediatric Disorders

See Child Health and Safety for pediatric disorders and web sites of interest.

Physical Medicine and Rehabilitation

➤ American Academy of Physical Medicine and Rehabilitation
   http://www.aapmr.org

Information in the field of physical medicine and rehabilitation, care of patients with acute and chronic pain, musculoskeletal problems like back and neck pain, tendonitis, pinched nerves and fibromyalgia. Also covers catastrophic events resulting in paraplegia, quadriplegia or traumatic brain injury as well as strokes, orthopedic injuries, or neurological disorders such as multiple sclerosis, polio, or amyotropic lateral sclerosis (ALS). Consumer, public, and patient information, what's new, and a search site are provided.

➤ American Physical Therapy Association
   http://www.apta.org

Physical therapy information, publications and other resources are provided.

Physicians and Professional Organizations

➤ American Medical Association
    http://www.ama-assn.org

Information on physicians and their professional organizations in the United States.

➤ Healthfinder
    http://www.healthfinder.gov

Go to Professional Organizations for information desired.

Planned Parenthood
http://www.plannedparenthood.org

Provides information on sexual health, research, responsible choices, contraception, emergency contraception, legislative update, news archive and newsletter archive for teenagers and others.

Podiatry and Foot Disorders

See Musculoskeletal and Orthopedic Disorders for appropriate resources and Web sites.

Practice Guidelines (Clinical)

➤ American College of Cardiology
    http://www.acc.org

Clinical practice guidelines for various cardiovascular disorders.

➤ American College of Physicians/American Society of Internal Medicine
http://www.asim.org
http://www.acponline.org

Clinical practice guidelines for disorders within the scope of internal medicine. Go to Patient Care, then to Clinical Practice Guidelines. Click on Current Guidelines Update (after 1994), etc.

➤ American Heart Association
http://www.americanheart.org

Clinical Practice Guidelines for various cardiovascular diseases.

➤ American Medical Association
http://www.ama-assn.org

Variety of Clinical Practice Guidelines available. Go to Health Information, then to Patients, then to Medical Library and search under Medem for Clinical Practice Guidelines for managing and treating various diseases and conditions. Scroll down and click on to one(s) of interest.

➤ Center for Disease Control and Prevention
http://www.cdc.gov

Provides an extensive list of clinical practice guidelines. Go to CDC Prevention Guidelines and scroll down list for recommended ways to prevent or treat a given disease or condition.

➤ National Guideline Clearinghouse
http://www.guideline.gov

Collaborative effort of American Medical Association, US Department of Health and Human Services, and American Association of Health Plans. This site contains practice guidelines from government and professional organizations. Use search site provided to obtain guideline information.

Preventive Medicine

➤ American College of Preventive Medicine
  http://www.acpm.org
  http://www.acpm.org/links.htm
  http://www.acpm.org/adult.htm

National medical specialty group of physicians dedicated to disease prevention and health and wellness promotion. Click on Preventive Medicine Resource Center for information on:

- Adolescent health
- Aging
- Cancer
- Clinical preventive services
- Consumer safety
- Disease prevention
- Health promotion
- Health statistics
- HIV and AIDS
- Immunization
- Infectious disease
- Injury prevention
- Managed care
- Maternal and child health
- Mental health
- Nutrition

- Occupational and environmental medicine
- Preventive medicine
- Public health
- Research
- Substance abuse
- Tobacco
- Wellness
- Women's health

Other related medical associations, health care sites, government agencies, and other sites and publications are highlighted.

Click on Adult Immunization for policy statement and evidence of effectiveness of the influenza, measles/mumps/rubella, pneumococcal pneumonia and tetanus/ diptheria toxoid vaccines. Advisory Committee on Immunization Practices recommendations for immunizations are provided. Sites for additional information are provided for:

- Cervical cancer screening
- Childhood immunization
- Screening symptomatic women for ovarian cancer
- Screening for prostate cancer
- Screening for skin cancer
- Screening mammography for breast cancer
- Skin protection from ultraviolet light exposure
- Tobacco cessation patient counseling

➤ American Society for Preventive Oncology
  http://www.aspo.org

Information regarding cancer prevention.

➤ Centers for Disease Control and Prevention

http://www.cdc.gov/health

Leading Federal effort for information on disease prevention and control.

➤ National Coalition on Healthcare
   http://www.americanshealth.org

Information regarding efforts to improve the nation's health.

Psychology and Counseling

➤ American Psychiatric Association
   http://www.psych.org/main.html

Go to diagnosis and treatment of mental and emotional illnesses and substance abuse disorders. Also go to APA Online Clinical Resources search site for additional information on psychology and counseling.

➤ Cyber Psych Link
   http://www.cyber-psych.com

Information and links regarding psychology and behavioral medicine along with a list of services and databases.

➤ Mental Health Net
   http://www.mentalhelp.net

One of the oldest and largest online mental health guide, community and provider of information on counseling services.

➤ Yahoo.com: Health: Counseling

http://www.dir.yahoo.com/Health/MentalHealth/Counseling_and
_Therapy/ Therapeutic_Methods

Categories featured include:

- Animal assisted therapy
- Arts therapy
- Biofeedback
- Client-centered therapy
- Clinics and practices
- Conferences
- Eye movement desensitization and reprocessing (EMDR)
- Gestalt therapy
- Group therapy
- Horticultural therapy
- Hypnosis
- Journals
- Narrative therapy
- Organizations
- Pastoral counseling
- Play therapy
- Primal psychotherapy
- Psychoanalysis
- Psychodrama
- School counseling
- Transactional analysis

Other sites on:

- Brief therapy center
- Ego analysis
- False memory syndrome information and resources

- Guide to psychotherapy
- Health psychology and rehabilitation
- International evaluation counseling communities
- Liberation psychotherapy
- Psychotherapy
- Working therapeutically with self and system

Antipsychiatry sites include:

- Antipsychiatry coalition: articles stating arguments against psychiatry
- Antipsychiatry reading room: with drug information, personal experience and more
- Ban shock therapy; opposing vies on shock therapy
- Center for the study of psychiatry and psychology: critique of value of psychiatry and psychology
- Citizen's commission on human rights: organization dedicated to exposing and eradicating criminal acts and human rights abuses by psychiatry
- Citizens for higher ethical standards in medicine: concerned about the abuse of human rights by psychiatry
- Lunatics liberation front: information network whose main subject is alternatives to psychiatry
- Psych.crime: reporting fraud, malpractice and sexual abuse by psychiatrists
- Support coalition international: for psychiatric survivors

Public Health and Consumer Medicine

➢ American Medical Association
http://www.ama-assn.org/consumer/gnrl.htm

Leading resource for consumer medicine.

➢ Medlineplus
  http://www.nlm.nih.gov/medlineplus

National Library of Medicine resource for public/consumer medicine information.

➢ PubMed
  http://www.ncbi.nlm.nih.gov/pubmed

PubMed is the National Library of Medicine's search service that includes over 10 million citations on Medline, PreMedline and other related databases, with links to participating online journals on almost any health topic of interest. Allows you to search public medicine topics of interest for free.

Radiology

➢ American College of Radiology
  http://www.acr.org

Radiology, services, links and search capability are provided.

➢ American Society for Therapeutic Radiology and Oncology
  http://www.astro.org

Radiation therapy for prostate cancer, breast cancer, etc., are available along with related health links.

Rare Disorders

➢ National Institutes of Health Office of Rare Diseases
  http://www.rarediseases.info.nih.gov

Information on more than 6,000 rare diseases, including current research, publications from scientific and medical journals, completed research, ongoing studies and patient support groups/links.

Reproductive Medicine

➤ American College of Obstetrics and Gynecology
http://www.acog.org

Search site for information of interest on reproductive medicine.

➤ American Society for Reproductive Medicine
http://www.asrm.org

Organization devoted to advancing knowledge and expertise in reproductive medicine. Information provided for patients, professionals, media, find a doctor and search the site for information on reproductive medicine topics of interests.

➤ Cornell University Center for Male Reproductive Medicine and Microsurgery
http://www.maleinfertility.org

New York Presbyterian Hospital and Weil Medical College of Cornell University offer effective new procedures and technologies available in infertility today with a high success rate. Search site provided for reproductive medicine topics of interest.

➤ Cornell University Center for Reproductive Medicine and Infertility
http://www.ivf.org

Google Web Directory: Health

➤ http://www.directory.google.com/top/health

Click on Reproductive Health for information of interest.

➤ Netscape: Health
http://www.health.netscape.com/health

Go to Health Search Categories and click on Reproductive Health.

➤ Yahoo: Health
http://dir.yahoo.com/health

Under Health Information, click on Reproductive Health

Sexually Transmitted Diseases

➤ Centers for Disease Control and Prevention
http://www.cdc.gov/health

Comprehensive information on sexually transmitted diseases.

➤ Duke University Healthy Devil Online
http://www.healthydevil.stuaff.duke.edu

Provides information on sexually transmitted diseases from the stand-point of university life.

➤ Intelihealth
http://www.intelihealth.com

Click on site for Sexual and Reproductive Health for information on sexually transmitted diseases.

➢ Google Web Directory: Health
   http://www.directory.google.com/top/health

Under Conditions and Diseases click on to Sexually Transmitted Diseases for information.

➢ National Institute of Allergy and Infectious Diseases
   http://www.niaid.nih.gov

Click on Infectious Diseases and search for Sexually Transmitted Diseases. Both the Centers for Disease Control and Prevention and the National Institute of Allergy and Infectious Diseases are leading US Government efforts regarding sexually transmitted disease.

➢ Web Crawler: Health
   http://www.webcrawler.com/health

Click on Sexual Health for information on Sexually Transmitted Disease.

Skin Disorders (Dermatology)

➢ American Academy of Dermatology
   http://www.aad.org

Provides access to SkinCarePhysicians.com which features current information on treatment and management of skin disease.

Also features sites for:
   • Acne Net
   • Dermatologist locator
   • *Journal American Academy Dermatology* online
   • Locating a free skin cancer screening facility near you

- Melanoma Net
- Patient information
- Professional information
- Sulzberger Institute for Dermatology

➤ American College of MOHS Micrographic Surgery and Cutaneous Oncology
   http://www.mohscollege.org

Features information on MOHS micrographic surgery as a specialized technique for the removal of skin cancer.

➤ American Society for Dermatologic Surgery
   http://www.asds-net.org

Promotes excellence in the subspecialty of dermatologic surgery. Features sites for:

- Finding a dermatologic surgeon (by name, state, or procedure/treatment)
- Methods to healthy skin and patient information pamphlets
- Other professional, academic, and non-profit web sites related to dermatologic surgery
- Overview of popular dermatologic treatments
- Procedures dermatologic surgeons perform along with before and after photos
- What's new, policy and issues

➤ National Institute of Arthritis and Musculoskeletal and Skin Diseases
   http://www.nih.gov/niams/healthinfo

Leading Federal effort providing information on skin disorders. Use search site for information on skin disorders topics of interest.

➤ National Psoriasis Foundation
  http://www.psoriasis.org

Resource for people who have psoriasis or psoriatic arthritis, their friends, family members, health care professionals, and the general public. A site is provided for you to search for further information on psoriasis or psoriatic arthritis topics of interest.

Sleep Disorders

➤ American Academy of Sleep Medicine
  http://www.aasmnet.org

Strives to increase awareness of sleep disorders in public and professional communities. Sites are provided for:
  • Association of Professional Sleep Society
  • Listing of Accredited Member Centers of Sleep Disorders Programs
  • Listing of the more commonly recognized sleep disorders sites
  • MED Sleep Educational Tools
  • Sleep
  • Sleep Hygiene Tips
  • Sleep Medicine Education and Research Foundation
  • Sleep Research Society
  • Why Can't I Sleep
  • Why Am I So Tired

➤ Medlineplus (Sleep Disorders)
  http://www.nlm.nih.gov/medlineplus/sleepdisorders.html

Search for sleep disorder information. Provides consumer and patient information on sleep disorders. Features sites with information provided in English or Spanish on the following topics:

- Alternative therapy
- Children's sleep disorders
- Clinical trials
- Coping with sleep disorders
- General aspects/overview of sleep disorders
- Medline search for recent articles on sleep disorders
- News
- Organizations involved in sleep disorders
- Search site for additional information on sleep disorders, drug information, dictionaries, directories and other resources
- Senior's sleep disorders
- Specific sleep disorders
- Treatment
- Women's sleep disorders

➢ National Center on Sleep Disorders Research
http://www.nhbli.nih.gov/about/nscdr/index.htm

Features information sites for:

- Additional Resources
- Links to Related Sites
- Publications
- Search sleep topic information
- Sleep and Driving in Youth
- Sleep Disorders

➢ National Sleep Foundation

http://www.sleepfoundation.org

Dedicated to prevention of accidents caused by sleep deprivation and excessive sleepiness and to enhanced quality of life for millions who suffer from sleep disorders. Sites provide information on:

- Drowsy Driving
- Insomnia
- Jet Lag
- Publications
- Parasomnias
- Periodic Limb Movement
- Narcolepsy
- Resource Links
- Restless Leg Syndrome
- Sleep Apnea
- Sleep Disorders
- Sleep Services and Resources
- What's New

Sports Medicine and Sports Disorders

➤ American College of Sports Medicine
http://www.acsm.org

Promotes and integrates scientific research and practical applications of sports medicine and exercise science to maintain and enhance physical performance, fitness, health and quality of life. Publications and search sites also are available.

Statistical Resources On the Web

➤ Centers for Disease Control and Prevention
  http://www.cdc.gov/health

Provides comprehensive statistics on diseases and conditions as well as leading causes of death.

➤ Statistical Resources on the Web (Health)
  http://lib.umich.edu/libhome/documents.center/sthealth.html

University of Michigan Documents Center features statistical health resources on the Web. A directory and search capability is provided. Categories of information featured include:

- Abortion
- Accidents
- AIDS
- Births
- Comprehensive
- Deaths and Death Index
- Disabilities
- Disease
- Experimentation
- Hazardous substances
- Health care
- Health insurance
- HMOs
- Hospitals
- International
- Life tables
- Mental health
- Noise
- Nursing homes

- Nutrition
- Pregnancy
- Prescription drugs
- Risk behaviors
- Sleep
- Social security
- Substance abuse
- Surgery
- Transplants
- Vital statistics

Stress

➢ American Institute of Stress
   http://www.stress.org

Dedicated to advancing knowledge regarding the role of stress in health and disease. Sites provided for information on:

- American's #1 Health Problem
- Expert Consultation
- Health Related Topics
- Information Packets on Stress
- Job Stress
- Monthly Newsletter
- Other networking links on Stress

➢ Google Web Directory: Health
   http://www.directory. google.com/top/health

Obtain stress related information from the Directory. Also search Stress and go to Links on Stress Related Resources for Stress Management and Emotional Wellness Links (http: //www.imt.net/~randolfi/stresslinks.html)

➤ Pub Med
   http://www.ncbi.nlm.nih.gov/pubmed

National Library of Medicine resource on stress and its prevention and treatment. Search for stress information

➤ StopStress.com
   http://www.stopstress.com

Features sites for information on:

> • Assessment
> • Holiday Stress
> • Humor and Stress
> • Occupational Stress
> • Relaxation Techniques
> • Stress Management
> • Treatment

➤ Web Crawler: Health
   http://www.webcrawler.com/health

Search for stress information and links.

Stroke

➤ American Heart Association
   http://www.americanheart.org

Use search site, etc. for pertinent stroke information.

➤ National Institute of Neurological Disorders
   http://www.ninds.nih.gov

Leading federal effort regarding stroke research prevention, and treatment. Search for information on stroke topics of interest.

Suicide and Prevention

➤ American Association of Suicidology
   http://www.suicidology.org

Organization dedicated to the understanding and prevention of suicide. Serves as a resource for anyone concerned about suicide: researchers, therapists, prevention specialists, survivors of suicide and people who are themselves in crisis. If you are currently in crisis, a site is provided to click onto for information on possible steps you can take to receive the help you need.

A "Report of the Committee on Physician Assisted Suicide and Euthanasia" is available.

Other sites are provided for information on:

- Available resources
- Contact AAS
- Conference info
- Crisis Center in Your Area
- Do You Need an Experienced Speaker About Suicide or Suicide Prevention
- Health links
- National Directory of Support Groups for Survivors of Suicide

- New Resources for Clinicians Who Have Lost a Patient to Suicide
- What's New

➤ American Psychiatric Association
   http://www.psych.org/main.html

Go to APA Online and search for information on suicide. Scroll down and click on suicide topics of interest.

➤ Centers for Disease Control and Prevention (Suicide)
   http://www.cdc.gov/health/violence.htm

Go to Health Topics A to Z and click on Violence/Suicide and then click on Suicide in the United States. CDC lists suicide as one of the 10 leading causes of death in America. Also go to National Center for Injury Prevention and Control at:
   http:// www.cdc.gov/ncipc/factsheets/suifacts.htm

Surgery

➤ American Academy of Facial Plastic and Reconstructive Surgery
   http://www.facial_plastic_surgery.org

Resource for information on plastic and reconstructive surgery.

➤ American Academy of Neurological and Orthopedic Surgeons
   http://www.aanos.org

Neurological and orthopedic surgery information.

➤ American Academy of Orthopedic Surgeons

http://www.aanos.org

Orthopedic surgery information.

➤ American Association of Neurological Surgeons
   http:// www. neurosurgery.org/aans

Neurological surgery information.

➤ American College of Mohs Micrographic Surgery and Cutaneous
   Oncology
   http://www.mohscollege.org

Facts about MOHS micrographic surgery and Find a MOHS Surgeon
sites are available

➤ American College of Surgeons
   http://www.facs.org

Features sites on:

> • Advocacy
> • *Journal of the American College of Surgeons*
> • Health policy
> • Library
> • Medline search topics of interest
> • Other Web sites of interest
> • Public information
> • Resources
> • Statements and guidelines
> • Surgical services

➤ American Society for Dermatologic Surgery
   http://www.asds_net.org
➤ American Society for Mohs Surgery
   http://www.skincancerinfo.com

➤ American Society for Surgery of the Hand
   http://www.hand_surgery.org

Hand surgery information.

➤ Your Surgery.com
   http://www.yoursurgery.com

Database synopsis of operative procedures designed to educate the average individual about their surgery. This site explains the most commonly performed surgeries using simple diagrams and cutting edge animation. Surgery of the head, neck, chest, abdomen, pelvis, back and limbs is covered. Each procedure described includes the following information:

- Alternative surgical options
- Anatomy of the area in which operation is performed
- Description (concise) of each surgery and associated ailment
- Innovations in surgical techniques
- Methods of diagnosis
- Pathology of the illness
- Possible complications of surgery
- Post operative care

You may receive notice of new surgical procedures. Click on to Related Surgical Sites for additional surgery information.

Transplantation

➤ International Society for Heart and Lung Transplantation
  http://www.ishlt.org

  Provides general transplant information and:

  > • Annual Transplant Registry
  > • Board and committee information
  > • Heart Failure Registry
  > • Programs and services
  > • Transplant notification entry

➤ National Institute of Allergy and Infectious Diseases
  http://www.niaid.nih.gov

  Current information on immunology and transplantation. Use search site to obtain further transplantation information of interest.

➤ National Institutes of Health Institutes and Centers
  http://www.nih.gov.icd

  Go to the appropriate NIH Institute and click on transplantation information regarding a particular organ system involved (i.e., heart, lung, kidneys, liver, etc.).

Travel Health

➤ Centers for Disease Control and Prevention: Travel Information Page
  http://www.cdc.gov/travel

Click on Traveler's Health and choose a topic(s) for information of interest. For the most recent health and travel developments see the Blue Sheet updated monthly.

➤ Shoreland's Travel Health Online
    http://www.tripprep.com

Utilizes the widely recognized health information sources including the World Health Organization, US Centers for Disease Control and Prevention, US Department of State (USDOS), the Program for Monitoring Emerging Diseases (ProMed) and news media, and medical literature. Provides health and wellness tips, destination details, general travel health concerns, guidelines for pre-trip planning, pointers for travelers who have special health conditions and vaccination requirements. Covers various specialized topics and travel precautions, and what you should do if you pick up an illness which doesn't produce symptoms until you have returned home. Country summary profiles provides information on special health considerations for countries you plan to visit, immunization recommendations, disease risk summaries, official health data and requirements and USDOS advisories.

Urological Disorders

➤ American Foundation for Urologic Disease
    http://www.prostatehealth.com
    http://www.afud.org/home.html

Information on prostate disease and other urological disorders.

➤ American Urological Association
    http://www.auanet.org

Information and publications about urological disease and conditions. Search site provided for further information on urological disorders.

➤ National Association for Incontinence
http://www.nafc.org

Dedicated to improving the quality of life of people with incontinence. Education, advocacy and support to the public and health professionals about the causes, prevention, diagnosis, treatments and management alternatives for incontinence. Publications include: *Quality Care*, a quarterly newsletter that provides moral support and practical information, *Resource Guide*, provides information on products which may be helpful for different types of incontinence, as well as pamphlets, audiovisuals, and books designed to educate the general public and health care professionals are provided

➤ National Institute of Diabetes, Digestive and Kidney Diseases
http://www.niddk.nih.gov

Leading Federal effort on kidney and other urological disorders. You may use search site provided to obtain information on urological disorders of interest.

➤ Prostateinfo.com
http://www.prostateinfo.com

A variety of information on prostate disease including PSA test, Gleason grading system, and more about benign prostatic hypertropy and prostate cancer.

Vaccines and Immunization Schedules

➢ American Academy of Family Physicians
  http://www.aafp.org

Provides vaccine information and recommended immunization schedules in children and adults

➢ American College of Preventive Medicine (Adult Immunizations)
  http://www.acpm.org/adult.htm

Click on Preventive Medicine Resource Center and go to site on Immunization for information/recommendations

➢ American Medical Association
  http://www.ama-assn.org

Use search site to obtain latest information on vaccines and immunization schedules in children and adults.

➢ Centers for Disease Control and Prevention (Health)
  http://www.cdc.gov/health

Provides comprehensive information on immunizations. Click on Traveler's Health for travel immunization precautions.

➢ Shoreland's Travel Health Online
  http://www.tripprep.com

Provides information on special health considerations for countries and places you plan to visit, immunization recommendations, disease risk summaries, official health data, and requirements and advisories.

Veteran's Health
http://www.va.org

Provides information on VA programs and veterans health, benefits and facilities worldwide.

Violence Prevention

➢ American College of Obstetricians and Gynecologists
http://www.acog.org

Go to Violence Against Women for information.

➢ Centers for Disease Control and Prevention
http://www.cdc.gov/health/violence.htm

Comprehensive US Government effort on violence prevention. Go to Health Topics A to Z and click on Violence and Suicide. Sites featured include:

- American Indian/Alaska Natives and Intimate Partner Violence
- Dating Violence
- Domestic Violence
- Firearm-Related Injuries
- Intimate Partner Violence
- Male Batterers
- Sexual Violence Against People with Disabilities
- Suicide in the United States
- Co-occurrence of Intimate Partner Violence Against Mothers and Abuse of Children
- Violence in the Workplace

- Violence and Reproductive Health
- Youth Violence

Vitamins

➤ American Academy of Family Physicians
  http://www.aafp.org

Go to Consumer Health and click on Supplements, Herbs or Vitamins for available information. Use site provided to search for further information of interest on vitamins.

➤ American College of Preventive Medicine
  http://www.acpm.org

Use site provided to search for preventive medicine health benefits of vitamins.

➤ American Medical Association
  http://www.ama-assn.org

Go to Consumer Health Information and click on site for Vitamins.

➤ Intellihealth
  http://www.intellihealth.com

Go to Intellihealth Home and click on site for Vitamins.

➤ Medlineplus (Vitamins)
  http://www.nlm.nih.gov/medlineplus/vitamins

Search for information on vitamins of interest or in general.

➤ PubMed (National Library of Medicine)
  http://ncbi.nlm.nih.gov/pubmed

Search for currently available information of interest on vitamins.

Wellness

➤ National Wellness Institute
  http://www.nationalwellness.org

International non-profit, professional membership organization established to meet the growing need of professionals engaged in wellness and health. Provides a wide variety of wellness information of interest.

➤ Net Wellness
  http://www.netwellness.org

Consumer quality health and wellness information and education services created and evaluated by the faculty of the University of Cincinatti, the Ohio State University, and Case Western Reserve University. Features sites on:

- About wellness
- Ask an expert
- Clinical trials
- Health centers
- Health topics
- How to use the information
- Library
- Referrals/directories
- Search wellness topics of interest
- What's new

➢ Wellness Web
  http://www.wellbweb.com

  See Search Engines, Directories, and Index section for information offered.

Women's Health

➢ American College of Obstetricians and Gynecologists
  http://www.acog.org

  Features sites for:

> • Adolescent care
> • Find a physician
> • Journal of Obstetrics and Gynecology
> • Managing menopause
> • Other information
> • Patient and professional education
> • Publications
> • Violence against women
> • Women's issues

➢ American Medical Association (Women's Health Information Center)
  http://www.ama-assn.org/special/womh/womh.htm

  Covers women's diseases, conditions and issues.

➢ American Medical Women's Association
  http://www.amwa-doc.org/index.html

  Information on women's issues, diseases and conditions

➤ British Medical Journal (Collections)
http://www.bmj.com/collections

Contains full text articles, editorials and reviews from 1998 to present in several areas of women's health including pregnancy, family planning, reproductive medicine, menopause, cervical cancer screening, oncology, incontinence and obstetrics and gynecology.

➤ Doctor's Guide to the Internet (Menopause)
http://www.pslgroup.com/menopause

Menopause related information and resources.

➤ Komen Breast Cancer Foundation
http://www.komen.org

Specializes in breast disease/cancers current information.

➤ National Guideline Clearinghouse
http://www.guideline.gov

Collaborative effort of AMA, the US Department of Health and Human Services and the American Association of Health Plans. This site contains practice guidelines concerning women's health from government and professional organizations. Enter the word "women" in their search site to obtain screening guidelines for conditions ranging from breast cancer and osteoporosis to sexually transmitted diseases.

➤ National Women's Health Information Center
http://www.4women.org

Comprehensive resource for women's health information.

➤ National Women's Health Resource Center
   http://www.healthywomen.org

Resource for a variety of women's health information.

➤ North American Menopause Society
   http://www.menopause.org

Extensive information on female menopause and its treatment.

➤ Society for Advancement of Women's Health Research
   http://www.women's_health.org

Information on issues in women's health research and links to groups with a specific disease focus.

➤ Women's Health Matters
   http://www.womenshealthmatters.ca

Sponsored by State University of New York Woman's College Health Sciences Center and Center for Research in Women's Health of Canada affiliated with the University of Toronto, Canada. Source of evidence-based information on women's health. Provides information on women's diseases, lifestyles, news and research findings

➤ Women's Health Resource Center (Mayo Clinic Health Oasis)
   http://www.mayohealth.org/mayo/common/htm/womenpg.htm

Provides extensive information on women's health issues, diseases, conditions and treatments. Alternative web site is http://www.mayohealth.org and click on Women under Centers for information on women's health.

Chapter VI

Health Resources and Web Sites

(Alphabetical List of 331 Resources and 372 Corresponding Web Sites)

All Web sites listed are proceeded with http://www. which
has been omitted in each instance for brevity and clarity.
For example, the Academy of Psychosomatic Medicine Web site
would be entered as http:// www. apm.org

Resources and Web Site

Academy of Psychosomatic Medicine
> **apm.org**

Achoo Gateway to Healthcare (Human Health and Disease Directory
> **achoo.com/directory/hhd/diseases.asp**

Agency for Healthcare Research and Quality
> **ahrq.gov**
> **ahrq.gov/consumer/20tips.htm**
> **ahrq.gov/qual/errors.htm**

Alcoholics Anonymous
> **alcoholics-anonymous.org**

All the Web, All the Time (Search)
> **alltheweb.com**

Alta Vista
> **altavista.com**

Alta Vista: Health Web Directory
> **dr.altavista.com/top/health**

Alternative Medicine Homepage
> **pitt.edu/~cbw.altm.html**

Alzheimers.com
> **alzheimers.com**

Alzheimer's Disease Education and Referral Center
> **alzheimers.org/adear**

Alzheimer's Research Foundation
> **alzheimers_research.org**

America on Line
> **aol.com**

America On Line Web Center:Health
> **aol.com/webcenters/health/home.adp**

American Academy of Allergy, Asthma and Immunology
> **aaaai.org**

American Academy of Audiology
> **audiology.org**

American Academy for Cerebral Palsy and Developmental Medicine
> **aacpdm.org**

American Academy of Child and Adolescent Psychiatry
> **aacap.org**

American Academy of Clinical Psychiatrists
> **aacp.com**

American Academy of Dermatology
> **aad.org**

American Academy of Disability Evaluating Physicians
> **aadep.org/intro.htm**

American Academy of Facial Plastic   and Reconstructive Surgery
    facial_plastic_surgery.org
American Academy of Family Physicians
    aafp.org
    aafp.org/exam
American Academy of Head, Neck and Facial Pain
    aahnfp.org
American Academy of Hospice and Palliative Medicine
    aahpm.org
American Academy of Neurological and Orthopedic Surgeons
    aanos.org
American Academy of Neurological Surgeons
    neurosurgery.org/aans
American Academy of Neurology
    aan.com
American Academy of Ophthalmology
    eyenet.org
American Academy of Orthopedic Surgeons
    aaos.org
American Academy of Otolaryngic Allergy
    allergy_ent.org
American Academy of Otolaryngology
    entnet.org
    entnet.org/patient.html
American Academy of Pain Medicine
    painmed.org
American Academy of Pediatrics
    aap.org
American Academy of Periodontology
    perio.org
American Academy of Physical Medicine and Rehabilitation
    aapmr.org

American Academy of Sleep Medicine
> **aasmnet.org**

American Association of Immunologists
> **aai/default.asp**

American Association on Mental Retardation
> **aamr.org/index**

American Association of Neurological Surgeons
> **neurosurgery.org/aans**

American Association of Suicidology
> **suicidology.org**

American Autoimmune Related Diseases Association
> **aarda.org**

American Botanical Council
> **herbalgram.org**
> **herbalgram.org/commission_e/index.html**

American Cancer Society
> **cancer.org**

American Cleft Palate and Craniofacial Association
> **cleft.org**

American College of Allergy, Asthma and Immunology
> **allergy.mcg.edu**

American College of Cardiology
> **acc.org**

American College of Chest Physicians
> **chestnet.org**

American College of Gastroenterology
> **acg.gi.org**

American College of Medical Genetics
> **faseb.org/genetics/acmg/acmgmenu.htm**

American College of Mohs Micrographic Surgery and Cutaneous Oncology
> **mohscollege.org**

American College of Nutrition
am_coll_nutr.org
American College of Obstetrics and Gynecology
acog.org
American College Occupational and Environmental Medicine
acoem.org
American College of Preventive Medicine
acpm.org
acpm.org/links.htm
acpm.org/adult.htm
American College of Physicians/American Society of Internal Medicine
acponline.org
asim.org
American College of Radiology
acr.org
American College of Rheumatology
rheumatology.org/index.asp
American College of Sports Medicine
acsm.org
American College of Surgeons
facs.org
American Dental Association
ada.org
ada.org/tc-clin.html
American Diabetes Association
diabetes.org
American Dietetic Association
eatright.org
American Epilepsy Society
aesnet.org
American Foundation for the Blind
afb.org

American Foundation for Urologic Disease
afud.org/home.html
prostatehealth.com
American Gastroenterological Association
gastro.org
American Geriatric Society
americangeriatrics.org
American Heart Association
americanheart.org
americanheart.org/dietaryguidelines/index.html
American Hiking Society
americanhiking.org
American Industrial Hygiene Association
aiha.org
American Institute of Stress
stress.org
American Juvenile Arthritis Organization
arthritis.org/answers/about_ajao.asp
American Liver Foundation
liverfoundation.org
American Lung Association
lungusa.org
American Medical Association
ama-assn.org
American Medical Association (General Health Issues)
ama-assn.org/ consumer/gnrl.htm
American Medical Association (Guidelines)
ama-assn.org/ about/guidelines.htm
American Medical Association (Women's Health Information Center
ama-assn.org/special/womh/ womh.htm
American Medical Women's Association
amwa-doc.org/index.html

American Orthopedic Foot and Ankle Society
    aofas.org
American Pain Society
    ampainsoc.org
American Parkinsons Disease Association
    apdaparkinson.com
American Physical Therapy Association
    apta.org
American Podiatric Medical Association
    apma.org
American Psychiatric Association
    psych.org/main.html
American Psychoanalytic Association
    apsa.org
American Psychological Association
    helping.apa.org
    apa.org
American Psychosomatic Society
    psychosomatic.org
American Society for Clinical Nutrition
    faseb.org/ascn
American Society for Dermatologic Surgery
    asds-net.org
American Society for Gastrointestinal Endoscopy
    asge.org
American Society of Hematology
    hematology.org
American Society for Mohs Surgery
    skincancerinfo.com
American Society of Pediatric Hematology and Oncology
    aspho.org

American Society of Preventive Oncology
    aspo.org
American Society for Reproductive Medicine
    asrm.org
American Society for Surgery of the Hand
    hand_surgery.org
American Society for Therapeutic Radiology and Oncology
    astro.org
American Urological Association
    auanet.org
Americans Health
    americanshealth.org
Arthritis Foundation
    arthritis.org
Ask a Biologist
    askabiologist.asu.edu/research/seecolor/colortest.html
Association for Retarded Citizens (The ARC of the United States)
    thearc.org
Association of American Medical Colleges
    aamc.org
Asthma and Allergy Foundation of America
    aafa.org
Back Pain Resource Center
    backpainreliefonline.com
Baylor College of Medicine (Huffington Center on Aging)
    bcm.tmc.edu/hcoa.hcoa
Bio Med Net
    bmn.com
Breast Cancer Research
    breast-cancer-research.com
British Medical Journal
    bmj.com

British Medical Journal Collections
     bmj.com/collections
Buying Medical Products Online
     fda.gov/oc/buyonline
Cancer Care
     cancercareinc.org
Center for Eating Disorders
     eatingdisorders.org
Center for Nutrition Policy Promotion (U.S. Department of Agriculture)
     usda.gov/cnpp
Center Watch Clinical Trials Listing Service
     centerwatch.com
Centers for Disease Control and Prevention (Health)
     cdc.gov
     cdc.gov/health
Centers for Disease Control and Prevention (National Center for Injury Prevention and Control)
     cdc.gov/ncipc/factsheets/ suifacts.htm
Centers for Disease Control and Prevention: Travel Information Page
     cdc.gov/travel
Centers for Disease Control and Prevention (Violence)
     cdc.gov/health/violence.htm
Colds and Flu
     4colds4anything.com
     4flu4anything.com
Colorblindness
     healthlink.us.com/color-blindness.htm
     askabiologist.asu.edu/research/seecolor/colortest.html
     directory.google.com/top.health
Cornell University Center for Male Reproductive Medicine and Microsurgery
     maleinfertility.org

Cornell University Center for Reproductive Medicine and Infertility
ivf.org
Crohn's and Colitis Foundation of America
ccfa.org
CyberDiet
cyberdiet.com
CyberPsychLink
cyber_psych.com
Dartmouth Atlas of Health Care
dartmouthatlas.org
Death and Dying
death_dying.com/terminalillness
death_dying.com/gentle/planner.html
Depression.com
depression.com
Diabetes.com
diabetes.com
Diabetes Control Center
dr_diabetes.com
Dietary Guidelines: Revision 2000
americanheart.org/dietaryguidelines/index.html
Digestive Health Resource Center
gastro.org/public/digestinfo.html
Disabilities
directory.google.com/top/health
Doctor's Guide to the Internet
pslgroup.com
pslgroup.com/docguide.htm
Doctor's Guide to the Internet (Diabetes)
pslgroup.com/diabetes
Doctor's Guide to the Internet (Meditation)
pslgroup.com/meditation

Doctor's Guide to the Internet (Menopause)
pslgroup.com/menopause
Dr. Greene.com
drgreene.com
Dr. Koop.com
drkoop.com/health
Drug Info Net
druginfonet.com
Duke University Healthy Devil Online
healthydevil.stuaff.duke.edu
e-fit: (Online Health and Fitness Network)
efit.com
efit.com/basics
Endocrine Society
endo-society.org
Epilepsy.com
epilepsy.com
Excite Health
excite.com/health
Family Meds.com
familymeds.com
Fast Search
alltheweb.com
fastsearch.com
First Government
firtstgov.gov
firstgov.gov/topics/healthy.html
Fitness Center
justmove.org/home.cfm
Fitness Link
fitnesslink.com

Fitness at Women.com
> **women.com/fitness**

Food and Drug Administration
> **fda.gov**
> **fda.gov/oc/buyonline**
> **fda.gov/medwatch**

Food and Health Communications
> **foodandhealth.com**

Food Safety.Gov
> **foodsafety.gov**

Forest Service
> **fs.fed.us**

Gerontological Society of America
> **geron.org**

Glaucoma Research Foundation
> **glaucoma.org/glaucoma/html**

Global Fitness and Health
> **global_fitness.com**

Google
> **google.com**

Google Web Directory: Health
> **directory.google.com/ top/health**
> **directory.google.com/ top/health/medicine**
> **directory.google.com/top /health/medical_specialties**

Great Outdoors Recreation Pages
> **gorp.com**

Harvard Health Publications
> **health.harvard.edu/newsletters**

Harvard Medical Web
> **med.harvard.edu**

Harvard School of Dental Medicine
> **hsdm.med.harvard.edu**

Headache.com
>   **headache.com.au**

Headache.Net
>   **headache.net/html/netscape.html**

Health Answers
>   **healthanswers.com**

Health Directory
>   **healthdirectory.com**

Healthfinder
>   **healthfinder.gov**

Health Gate
>   **healthgate.com**

Health on the Net Foundation (Geneva, Switzerland)
>   **hon.ch**

Healthy People 2010
>   **health.gov/healthypeople/prevagenda.focus.htm**

Hepatitis Foundation International
>   **hepfi.org**

Hospice Net
>   **hospicenet.org**

Hotbot
>   **hotbot.com**

HotBot Directory: Health
>   **dir.hotbot.lycos.com/health**

Infoseek/Go
>   **infoseek.go.com**

Infoseek: Health and Wellness
>   **infoseek.go.com/center/healthgo.com/webdir/health**

Institute of Medicine (National Academy of Sciences)
>   **iom.edu**

Intelihealth
>   **intelihealth.com**

Interactive Healthy Eating Index
    usda.gov.cnpp
International Food and Information Council
    ifcinfo.health.org
International Foundation for Functional Gastrointestinal Disorders
    iffgd.org
International Society for Heart and Lung Transplantation
    ishlt.org
International Society of Refractive Surgery
    isrs.org
Internet Hospital Directory
    ds.dial.pipex.com/r.bowyer/hospital.html
Internet Medical School Directory
    ds.dial.pipex.com/r.bowyer/med_schl.htm
Internet Mental Health
    mentalhealth.com
Istituto Mario Negri (Milan, Italy)
    irfmn.mnegri.it
Karolinska Institutet (Stockholm, Sweden)
    mic.ki.se/diseases/index.html
Journal of American Medical Association
    jama.ama-assn.org
Kid's Health
    kidshealth.org
Komen Breast Cancer Foundation
    komen.org
Lancet
    thelancet.com
Learn the Net
    learnthenet.com
Learning Meditation Home Page
    learningmeditation.com

Leukemia and Lymphoma Society
> **leukemia_lymphoma.org**

Librarians' Index to the Internet
> **lii.org**

Life Clinic.com
> **lifeclinic.com**

Lighthouse International
> **lighthouse.org**

Looksmart
> **looksmart.com**

Looksmart: Health
> **looksmart.com/health**

Lycos
> **lycos.com**

Lycos Directory: Health
> **dir.lycos.com/health**

Magellan Health
> **magellan.excite.com/health**

Mayo Clinic Health Oasis
> **mayohealth.org**

MD Consult
> **mdconsult.com**

Med Explorer
> **medexplorer.com**

Med Help International
> **medhelp.org/home.htm**

Medical Matrix
> **medicalmatrix.org**

Medicine Net
> **medicinenet.com**

Mediconsult Health Network
> **mediconsult.com**

Meditation
>   **health.yahoo.com**
>   **mediation.com**

Medline (National Library of Medicine)
>   **nlm.nih.gov/medline**

Medlineplus
>   **nlm.nih.gov/medlineplus**

Medlineplus (Arthritis)
>   **nlm.nih.gov/medlineplus/arthritis.html**

Medlineplus (Meditation)
>   **nlm.nih.gov/medlineplus/meditation**

Medlineplus (National Library of Medicine)
>   **nlm.nih.gov/medlineplus**

Medlineplus (Sleep Disorders)
>   **nlm.nih.gov/medlineplus/sleepdisorders**

Medlineplus (Vitamins)
>   **nlm.nih.gov/medlineplus/vitamins**

Medscape
>   **medscape.com**

Med Web (Emory University Health Science)
>   **medweb.emory.edu/medweb**

Mental Health Net
>   **mentalhelp.net**

Merck Manual
>   **merck.com/pubs/mmanual**

MSN
>   **msn.com**
>   **health.msn.com**

Muscular Dystrophy Association
>   **mdausa.org**

National Academy for Child Development
>   **nacd.org**

National Academy of Sciences
 nas.edu
National Acupuncture and Oriental Medicine Alliance
 acuall.org
National Alliance for the Mentally Ill
 nami.org
National Association for Incontinence
 nafc.org
National Association for Down Syndrome
 nads.org
National Cancer Institute
 nci.nih.gov
National Center for Chronic Disease Prevention and Health Promotion
 cdc.gov/nccdphp/phyactive.htm
 cdc.gov/nccdphp/nutrisk.htm
 cdc.gov/nccdphp/sgr/mm.htm
 cdc.gov/nccdphp/tobacco.htm
National Center for Complimentary and Alternative Medicine
 nccam.nih.gov
National Center for Injury Prevention and Control
 cdc.gov/ncipc/factsheets.suifacts.htm
National Center on Sleep Disorders Research
 nhlbi.nih.gov/about/ncsdr/index.htm
National Chronic Fatigue and Fibromyalgia Association
 cfidsfoundation.org
National Coalition on Healthcare
 americashealth.org
National Council on Alcoholism and Drug Dependence
 ncadd.net
National Down Syndrome Society
 ndss.org

National Eye Institute
    nei.nih.gov
National Guideline Clearinghouse
    guideline.gov
National Headache Foundation
    headaches.org
National Heart, Lung and Blood Institute
    nhlbi.nih.gov
National Heart, Lung and Blood Institute: Health Information
    http://www.nhlbi.nih.gov
    nhlbi.nih.gov/health/public/heart/index.htm
    nhlbi.nih.gov/health/prof/heart/index.htm
    nhlbi.nih.gov/health/public/lung/index.htm
    nhlbi.nih.gov/health/prof/lung/index.htm
    nhlbi.nih.gov/health/public/blood/index.htm
National Human Genome Research Institute
    nhgri.nih.gov/index.html
National Institute on Aging
    nih.gov/nia
National Institute on Alcohol Abuse and Alcoholism
    niaaa.nih.gov
National Institute of Allergy and Infectious Disease
    niaid.nih.gov
National Institute of Arthritis and Musculoskelatal and Skin Diseases
    nih.gov/niams
    nih.gov/niams/healthinfo.gov
National Institute of Child Health and Human Development
    nichd.nih.gov
National Institute on Deafness and Other Communication Disorders
    nih.gov/nidcd
National Institute of Dental and Craniofacial Research
    nidcr.nih.gov/cranio/disease/ac.html

nidcr.nih.gov/news/publica.htm
National Institute of Diabetes and Digestive and Kidney Diseases
    niddk.nih.gov
National Institute on Drug Abuse
    nida.nih.gov
National Institute of Environmental Health Sciences
    niehs.nih.gov
National Institute of Health: Health Information
    nih.gov/health
National Institutes of Health Institutes and Centers
    nih.gov.icd
National Institute of Health Office of Rare Diseases
    rarediseases.info.nih.gov
National Institute of Mental Health
    nimh.nih.gov
National Institute of Neurological Disorders and Stroke
    ninds.nih.gov
National Institute of Health Clinical Center
    cc.nih.gov
    clinicalstudies.info.nih.gov
National Kidney Foundation
    kidney.org
National Library of Medicine
    nlm.nih.gov
National Mental Health Association
    nmha.org
National Multiple Sclerosis Society
    nmss.org
National Network of Libraries of Medicine
    nnlm.nlm.nih.gov/psr
National Osteoporosis Foundation
    nof.org

National Park Service
>**nps.gov**

National Parkinson Foundation
>**parkinson.org**

National Psoriasis Foundation
>**psoriasis.org**

National Senior Citizens Law Center
>**nsclc.org**

National Sleep Foundation
>**sleepfoundation.org**

National Wellness Institute
>**nationalwellness.org**

National Women's Health Information Center
>**4women.org**

National Women's Health Resource Center
>**healthywomen.org**

Natural Medicines Comprehensive Database
>**naturaldatabase.com**

NBCi.com: Health
>**nbci.com/directory/health**

Net Wellness
>**netwellness.org**

Netscape
>**netscape.com**

Netscape: Health
>**health.netscape.com/health/main.tmpl**

Netscape: Search Category Health
>**search.netscape.com/health**

New England Journal of Medicine
>**nejm.org**

North American Menopause Society
>**menopause.org**

Northern Light
>	**northernlight.com**

Office of Rare Diseases (National Institute of Health)
>	**raredisease.info.nih.gov/ord**

Occupational Safety and Health Administration (U.S. Department of Labor)
>	**osha.gov/safelinks.html**

Oncolink (University of Pennsylvania School of Medicine Cancer Center)
>	**oncolink.upenn.edu**

Outdoors.org
>	**outdoors.org**

Pain.com
>	**pain.com**

Pharmaceutical Information Net0work
>	**pharminfo.com**

Planned Parenthood Association
>	**plannedparenthood.org**

Planet Rx.com
>	**planetrx.com**

Prostateinfo.com
>	**prostateinfo.com**

Pub Med (National Library of Medicine)
>	**ncbi.nlm.nih.gov/pubmed**
>	**ncbi.nlm.nih.gov/pubmed/meshbrowserhelp.html**

Rational Recovery Systems
>	**rational.org/recovery**

Recommended Meta Search Tools (University of California at Berkley)
>	**lib.berkley.edu/TeachingLib/Guides/Internet/MetaSearch.html**

Recommended Search Engines (University of California at Berkeley)
>	**lib.berkeley.edu/TeachingLib/Guides/Internet/Search_Engines.html**

Recommended Search Tools (National network of Libraries of Medicine)
>	**nnlm.nlm.nih.gov/psr**

Recommended Search Tools (Search Engine Databases and Newswires)
Internets.com
Recommended Search Tools (University of California at Berkley)
lib.berkley.edu/TeachingLib/Guides/Internet/ToolsTables.html
Recommended Subject Directories (University of California at Berkeley)
lib.berkeley.edu/TeachingLib/Guides/Internet/SubjDirectories.html
Recreation.gov
recreation.gov
Rx List (The Internet Drug Index)
rxlist.com
Search Clinical Research Studies Database
clinicalstudies.info.nih.gov
Search Engine Databases and Newswires
internets.com
Search Engines
searchengines.com/search_engines.101.html
Shape Up America
shapeup.org
Shoreland's Travel Health Online
tripprep.com
Sleep Disorders Research Center (National Institutes of Health)
nhlbi.nih.gov/health/prof/sleep/index.htm
nhlbi.nih.gov/health/public/sleep/index.htm
Society for Adolescent Medicine
adolescenthealth.org
Society for Clinical and Experimental Hypnosis
sunsite.utk.edu/IJCEH/scehframe.htm
Society for the Advancement of Women's Health Research
womens_health.org
Society of General Internal Medicine
sgim.org

Society of Nuclear Medicine
> **snm.org**

Spine Health (Back Pain)
> **spine_health.com**

Statistical Resources on the Web (Health)
> **lib.umich.edu/libhome/documents.center/sthealth.html**

Stop Stress.com
> **stopstress.com**

Stress Management and Emotional Wellness Links
> **imt.net/~randolfi/stresslinks.html**

Symphony Group
> **thesymphonygroup.com**

Take Off Pounds Sensibly
> **tops.org**

Thyroid Foundation of America
> **tsh.org/main.html**

Tufts University Nutritional Navigator
> **navigator.tufts.ed**

United Cerebral Palsy Association
> **ucpa.org**

University of Hertfordshire (Hertfordshire, United Kingdom)
> **herts.ac.uk**
> **herts.ac.uk/lis/subjects/health/hlthwww.htm**

University of Maryland School of Medicine (Thoracic Surgery Division)
> **umm.edu/thoracic**

US Department of Agriculture (Nutrient Data Laboratory)
> **nal.usda.gov/fnic/foodcomp**

U.S. Forrest Service
> **fs/fed/us**

U.S. Pharmacopoeia
> **usp.org/body.htm**

Vegetarian Resource Group
> **vrg.org**

Verified Internet Pharmacy Practice Sites
> **nabp.net/vipps/intro.asp**

Veterans Affairs
> **va.org**

Web Crawler: Health
> **webcrawler.com**
> **webcrawler.com/health**

Web MD
> **shn.webmd.com**

Weights Net
> **weightsnet.com**

Wellness Web
> **wellweb.com**

Women's Health Matters Network
> **womenshealthmatters.ca**

Women's Health Resource Center (Mayo Clinic Health Oasis)
> **mayohealth.org/mayo/common/htm/womenpg.htm**

Yahoo: Health
> **dir.yahoo.com/health**
> **dir.yahoo.com/health/diseases_and_conditions**
> **dir.yahoo.com/health/web_directories**
> **dir.yahoo.com/health/mentalhealth/counseling_and_therapy/therapeutic_methods**

Yahoo Health (Counseling)
> **dir.yahoo.com/health/mental_health/counseling_and_therapy/therapeutic_methods**

Your Surgery.com
> **yoursurgery.com**

Chapter VII

Search the Internet/Web for Health Information

With your computer you are in a position to answer many, if not all, your health, wellness, and healthcare, questions at home at any time of the day or week via the Internet and Web. Many books have been written on how to use the Internet and Web. You can obtain one or more of these books for use from your local public library if you don't own one already. Use the latest edition available whenever possible.

A number of commercial services such as AOL, MSN, Netscape, Yahoo and others offer easy, reliable and relatively inexpensive access to the Web and even provide help using it. Use the one(s) of your own preference.

If you do not have a computer of your own, you can use a computer at your local public library to connect to the Internet and Web at no cost to you. And your librarian can show you not only how to connect to the Internet and Web but also instruct you in use. Also, you can employ a WebTV or similar device hooked up to your TV set at home to connect to the Internet and Web. Once you are connected to the Internet and Web, you are in a position to start searching.

Chapter III provides you with a number of Web Health Information Search Tools and corresponding Web Sites. Chapter IV highlights the

Author's List of Selected Useful SearchTools and Web Sites which you can use to start your search by topic. Select at least 3 search tools which appear to best suit your needs, taking into consideration information provided on each and compare healthcare information available. Chapters III and IV provide you with some useful suggestions for your consideration in searching. Each search tool reviewed enables you to search desired health information of interest using key words, topics or phrases. Most Web sties use colorful graphics and a hypertext or alternative search tool that allows you to click on to highlighted links which immediately shunts you to an additional source(s) of information. Chapter V is organized to provide information by Health Categories, Diseases, Resources and Web Sites. Health categories and diseases are listed alphabetically for ease of reference to obtain relevant resources and Web sites to expedite search for desired healthcare information.

There are three main types of health related resources on the Web. These are:

1) reference materials and information, 2) discussion and chat groups, and 3) expert consultation. Generally speaking, most useful are the reference materials and information, next the expert consultation and lastly the discussion and chat groups. Government and nonprofit professional organizations, hospital medical centers, medical schools and universities maintain Web sites which you can go to for reasonably reliable healthcare reference materials and information. Direct expert consultation also is available on the Web through select resources and sites. Discussion groups allow you to contact people and self help groups with similar problems but are not necessarily reliable. Selected commercial search tools discussed in this book also may offer useful information.

A reasonably broad spectrum of resources and Web sites is made available in Chapters III, IV, and V for obtaining information on almost any disease, condition or healthcare topic of interest. Chapter VI contains an alphabetical list of all resources and their corresponding Web sites referred to in this book. If you experience difficulty in reaching a particular Web site using the address (URL) provided, type in and search the resource name itself and this should bring you to the resource and Web page information desired.

Remember that the Web is growing rapidly daily and is in a constant state of flux. Search tools may change their resource names and Web sites. Alliances, formats, presentations, information offered and modus operandi also may change over time. Some may even merge or go out of business. If one search tool, resource, or Web site doesn't work for you, just try another from the list provided in Chapter VI.

Most, but not all, health, wellness, and healthcare information you find using the search tools, resources, and Web sites provided in this book likely will turn out to be reasonably useful in one way or another. However, you should not believe all health information you may find. Unlike articles published in peer reviewed professional journals, there is no guarantee that the Web information you obtain is current, accurate, or reliable. You should use caution regarding information obtained from those Web sites set up by commercial companies primarily to sell a product(s). Remember "buyer beware". Also, bear in mind that even the best of health Web sites may not be uniformly reliable in all areas covered, so compare and contrast results and consult with your physician or healthcare provider before reaching any conclusions.

Even in the case of evidence based health information, usually considered to be more reliable, there may be problems. Like all evidence, healthcare information is necessarily subject to interpretation and application. All of us are biased to some extent in one way or another in obtaining, interpreting and applying healthcare information, evidence based or not. Words, phrases, statistics, etc. mean different things to different people depending on "where they are coming from". For example, even with a long standing document such as the Constitution of the United States written by "great minds", people, lawyers, judges and even the Supreme court are still struggling to properly interpret and apply what the words, phrases, and sentences were meant to mean by our "founding fathers" who produced the document. Evidence based health information is no different in this regard: differences in interpretation and application still need to be considered.

One also needs to bear in mind that not all health and wellness information, or every treatment found on the Web is effective or safe, or even as effective as it is claimed to be: whether it is a health, wellness advice, or treatment such as a drug, surgical method, or a psychological or psychiatric therapy. That is why it has often been said in so many words "take the new treatment while it still works" and "today's therapeutics are tomorrow's witchcraft". Thus it is best to consider using health and wellness, or healthcare information obtained from the Web only in consultation with your physician or healthcare provider.

About the Author

Eugene A. DeFelice, M.D., is a widely acclaimed author, physician, educator, medical research scientist and distinguished Clinical Professor of Medicine at a leading U.S. Medical School. He is a Fellow of the American Geriatric Society and a Fellow of the Academy of Psychosomatic Medicine. Dr. DeFelice has received numerous honors and his biographical sketch is published in the Marquis Who's Who in America, Who's Who in the World, and Who's Who in Medicine and Healthcare. He has authored five previous books and published numerous medical and scientific articles in professional journals.

www.ingramcontent.com/pod-product-compliance
Lightning Source LLC
Chambersburg PA
CBHW061340280526
45784CB00001B/75